T0276638

Endocarditis: Causes, Treatments and Case Studies

Endocarditis: Causes, Treatments and Case Studies

Edited by **Jeff Wilson**

New Jersey

Published by Foster Academics,
61 Van Reypen Street,
Jersey City, NJ 07306, USA
www.fosteracademics.com

Endocarditis: Causes, Treatments and Case Studies
Edited by Jeff Wilson

International Standard Book Number: 978-1-63242-175-3 (Hardback)

Contents

Preface

In my initial years as a student, I used to run to the library at every possible instance to grab a book and learn something new. Books were my primary source of knowledge and I would not have come such a long way without all that I learnt from them. Thus, when I was approached to edit this book; I became understandably nostalgic. It was an absolute honor to be considered worthy of guiding the current generation as well as those to come. I put all my knowledge and hard work into making this book most beneficial for its readers.

The causes, treatments and case studies related to the disease of endocarditis are elucidated in this comprehensive book. Endocarditis is a disease that occurs as a result of inflammation of the endocardium. It is an inflammation of the inner lining of the heart (native or prosthetic valves). Endocarditis is characterized by a prototypic lesion, the vegetation, which is a mass of platelets, fibrin, microcolonies of microorganisms, and scant inflammatory cells. Structures such as the interventricular septum, tendinous chords, the mural endocardium or even intra-cardiac implants also get affected by it. The book presents the most prevalent causes and modern treatments of endocarditis, as well as cases where organs remote from the heart are affected by this disease.

I wish to thank my publisher for supporting me at every step. I would also like to thank all the authors who have contributed their researches in this book. I hope this book will be a valuable contribution to the progress of the field.

Editor

1

An Overview on Endocarditis

Breijo-Marquez and M. Pardo Rios
Commemorative Hospital, Boston, Massachusetts;
Catholic University, Murcia;
[1]USA
[2]Spain

1. Introduction

The endocardium is the innermost layer of tissue that lines the chambers of the heart. Its cells are embryologically and biologically similar to the endothelial cells that line blood vessels.

The endocardium underlies the much more voluminous myocardium, the muscular tissue responsible for the contraction of the heart. The outer layer of the heart is termed epicardium. Whole heart is surrounded by a small amount of fluid enclosed by a fibrous pouch called the pericardium.

Recently, it has become evident that the endocardium, which is primarily made up of endothelial cells, can have control over myocardial function. This modulating role is separate from the homeometric and heterometric regulatory mechanisms that control some myocardial contractility. Furthermore, the endothelium of the myocardial (heart muscle) and capillaries, which is also closely appositioned to the cardiomyocytes (heart muscle cells) are involved in this modulatory role. Thus, the cardiac endothelium (both the endocardial endothelium and the endothelium of the myocardial capillaries) controls the development of the heart in the embryo as well as in the adult, for example during cardiac hypertrophy. Additionally, the contractility and electrophysiological environment of the cardiomyocytes are regulated by the cardiac endothelium. This function recently known, it is extremely important to us when there are some injuries cardiac affecting to the myocardial infarction.

The endocardial endothelium may also act as a kind of blood-heart barrier (analogous to the blood-brain barrier), thus controlling the ionic composition of the extra-cellular fluid in which the cardiomyocytes bathe.

All inflammation of the endocardium is called, therefore, endocarditis.

Depending on how extensive of the inflammation, endocarditis can be: localized (most often) or generalized.

As in every inflammation, the cause of endocarditis can be infectious (virus, bacteria, parasites and so...) – bacteria is the most common - or non-infectious.

During depolarization, the impulse is carried from endocardium to epicardium, and during repolarization, the impulse moves from epicardium to endocardium. In infective endocarditis, the endocardium (especially the endocardium lining the heart valves) is affected by originating agent, (The majority, an infectious agent).

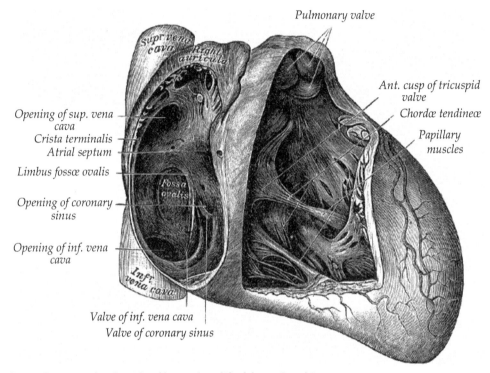

Fig. 1. Interior of right side of heart. (modified from Gray's)

Infective endocarditis is the most common form of endocarditis and its valves, the most affected structures, over all the mitral valve: The agents are usually bacterial, but other organisms can also be responsible.

The valves of the heart do not receive any dedicated blood supply. As a result, defensive immune mechanisms (such as white blood cells) cannot directly reach the valves via the bloodstream. If an organism (such as bacteria) attaches to valve surface and forms vegetation, the host immune response is blunted. The lack of blood supply to the valves also has implications on treatment, since drugs also have difficulty reaching the infected valve.

Normally, blood flows smoothly through these valves. If they have been damaged - from rheumatic fever, for example - the risk of bacterial attachment is increased.

Historically, infective endocarditis has been clinically divided into *acute* and subacute presentations (because untreated patients tended to livelonger with the subacute as opposed to the acute form). This classifies both the rate of progression and severity of disease.

Subacute bacterial endocarditis (SBE) is often due to streptococci of low virulence and mild to moderate disease, which progresses slowly over weeks and months and has low propensity to haematogenous seed extracardiac sites.

Acute bacterial endocarditis (ABE) is a fulminant infection over days to weeks, and is more likely due to Staphylococcus aureus which has much greater virulence, or disease-producing capacity and frequently causes metastatic infection. (Currently, the terms short incubation -meaning less than about six weeks-, and long incubation -greater than about six weeks- are preferred).

Infective endocarditis may also be classified as culture-positive or culture-negative. Culture-negative endocarditis can be due to micro-organisms that require a longer period of time to be identified in the laboratory, such organisms are said to be fastidious because they have demanding growth requirements, or due to absence of an organism as in marantic endocarditis. Some pathogens responsible for culture-negative endocarditis include Aspergillus species, Brucella species, Coxiella burnetii, Chlamydia species, and HACEK bacteria. Another possible reason for culture negativity, even with the more typical pathogens, is prior antibiotic treatment.

Endocarditis can also be classified by the side of the heart affected:

Patients who inject narcotics or other drugs intravenously may introduce infection, which will travel to the right side of the heart classically affecting the tricuspid valve, and most often caused by S. aureus.

In other patients without a history of intravenous exposure, endocarditis is more frequently left-sided. Another form of endocarditis is nosocomial endocarditis which is when the patient is diagnosed with endocarditis and has had hospital care one month prior to the incident and is usually secondary to IV catheters, Total parenteral nutrition lines, pacemakers, and so.

Besides, Endocarditis can have a classification according its affected valve types: The distinction between native-valve endocarditis and prosthetic-valve endocarditis is clinically important. Prosthetic valve endocarditis can be early (< 60 days of valvular surgery) or late (> 60 days of valvular surgery).

Early prosthetic-valve endocarditis is usually due to intraoperative contamination or a postoperative bacterial contamination, which is usually nosocomial in nature. Late prosthetic valve endocarditis is usually due to community acquired microorganisms.

In a healthy individual, a bacteraemia (where bacteria get into the blood stream through a minor cut or wound) would normally be cleared quickly with no adverse consequences. If a heart valve is damaged and covered with a piece of a blood clot, the valve provides a place for the bacteria to attach themselves and an infection can be established.

In the past, bacteremia caused by dental procedures (in most cases due to viridans streptococci, which reside in oral cavity), such as a cleaning or extraction of a tooth was thought to be more clinically significant than it actually was. However, it is important that a dentist or a dental hygienist be told of any heart problems before commencing treatment. Antibiotics are administered to patients with certain heart conditions as a precaution, although this practice has changed in the US, with new American Heart Association guidelines released in 2007, and in the UK as of March 2008 due to new NICE guidelines. Everyday tooth brushing and flossing will similarly cause bacteremia. Although there is little evidence to support antibiotic prophylaxis for dental treatment, the current American Heart Association guidelines are highly accepted by clinicians and patients.

Another group of causes results from a high number of bacteria getting into the bloodstream. Colorectal cancer (mostly Streptococcus bovis), serious urinary tract infections (mostly enterococci), and drug injection (*S. aureus*) can all introduce large numbers of bacteria. With a large number of bacteria, even a normal heart valve may be infected.

A more virulent organism (such as *S.* aureus, but see below for others) is usually responsible for infecting a normal valve.

Intravenous drug users tend to get their right-sided heart valves infected because the veins that are injected enter the right side of the heart, so they will have injured valves on that side that the bacteria can bind to. In rheumatic heart disease infection occurs on the aortic and the mitral valves, on the left side of the heart.

Other factors that increase the risk of developing infective endocarditis are low levels of white blood cells, immunodeficiency or immunosuppression, malignancy, diabetes, and alcohol abuse.

As we have already said, altered blood flow around the valves is a risk factor for obtaining endocarditis. The valves may be damaged congenitally, from surgery, from auto-immune mechanisms, or simply as a consequence of old age. The damaged part of a heart valve becomes covered with a blood clot, a condition known as non-bacterial thrombotic endocarditis (NBTE). Altered blood flow, and thus infective endocarditis, is more likely in high pressure areas.

Consequently, ventricular septal defects create more susceptibility than atrial septal defects. Damaged vascular endothelium will also promote platelet and fibrin deposition, upon which bacteria can take hold. Valvular lesions are a major cause of such damage, as are jet lesions resulting from ventricular septal defects or patent ductus arteriosus.

All patients should fulfill the Duke criteria in order to establish the diagnosis of endocarditis. As the Duke criteria rely heavily on the results of echocardiography, research has addressed when to order an echocardiogram by using signs and symptoms to predict occult endocarditis among patients with intravenous drug abuse and among non drug-abusing patients. Unfortunately, this research is over 20 years old and it is possible that changes in the epidemiology of endocarditis and bacteria such as staphylococci can make the following estimates incorrect.

2. Duke criteria

Established in 1994 by the Duke Endocarditis Society and revised in 2000, the Duke criteria are a collection of major and minor criteria used to establish a diagnosis of endocarditis. A diagnosis can be reached in any of three ways: two major criteria, one major and three minor criteria, or five minor criteria.

Major criteria include:

Positive blood culture with typical IE microorganism, defined as one of the following:

Typical microorganism consistent with IE from 2 separate blood cultures, as noted below:
Viridans-group streptococci, or
S. bovis including nutritional variant strains, or
HACEK group, or
S. aureus, or
Community-acquired enterococci, in the absence of a primary focus
Microorganisms consistent with IE from persistently positive blood cultures defined as:
Two positive cultures of blood samples drawn >12 hours apart, or
All of 3 or a majority of 4 separate cultures of blood (with first and last sample drawn 1 hour apart)
Coxiella burnetii detected by at least one positive blood culture or antiphase I IgG antibody titer >1:800
Evidence of endocardial involvement with positive echocardiogram defined as
Oscillating intracardiac mass on valve or supporting structures, in the path of regurgitant jets, or on implanted material in the absence of an alternative anatomic explanation, or
Abscess, or
New partial dehiscence of prosthetic valve or new valvular regurgitation (worsening or changing of pre-existing murmur not sufficient)

Minor criteria include:

Predisposing factor: known cardiac lesion, recreational drug injection
Fever >38°C
Evidence of embolism: arterial emboli, pulmonary infarcts, Janeway lesions, conjunctival hemorrhage
Immunological problems: glomerulonephritis, Osler's nodes
Positive blood culture (that doesn't meet a major criterion) or serologic evidence of infection with organism consistent with IE but not satisfying major criterion

High dose antibiotics are administered by the intravenous route to maximize diffusion of antibiotic molecules into vegetation(s) from the blood filling the chambers of the heart. This is necessary because neither the heart valves nor the vegetations adherent to them are supplied by blood vessels. Antibiotics are continued for a long time, typically two to six weeks. Specific drug regimens differ depending on the classification of the endocarditis as acute or subacute (acute necessitating treating for S. aureus with oxacillin or vancomycin in addition to gram-negative coverage). Fungal endocarditis requires specific anti-fungal treatment, such as amphotericin B. In acute endocarditis, due to the fulminant inflammation empirical antibiotic therapy is started immediately after the blood has been drawn for culture. This usually includes oxacillin and gentamicin IV infusions until the culture sensitivity report with the minimum inhibitory concentration comes, when the therapy can be modified to tailor to the microorganism.

There should be noted that the routine use of gentamicin to treat Staphylocococcal endocarditis has been questioned, given the lack of evidence to support its use and the high rate of complications.

In subacute endocarditis, antibiotic treatment is based on the micro organism involved, requiring the culture sensitivity report.

So immediate therapy is mainly focused on symptomatic treatment.

The most common organism responsible for infective endocarditis is viridans-group streptococci, which are highly sensitive to penicillin. High dose IV crystalline penicillin every 4hrs for 2 weeks is recommended and still remains the drug of choice.

Again it is important to note that antibiotic therapy hinges upon the culture sensitivity report.

The short course treatment in patients where the blood culture reveals the causative organism, culture sensitivity reports should be followed to treat the patient,

In addition to usage of two bactericidal antibiotics for a minimum of two weeks as a combination therapy.

Surgical debridement of infected material and replacement of the valve with a mechanical or bioprosthetic artificial heart valve is necessary in patients who fail to clear micro-organisms from their blood in response to antibiotic therapy, or in patients who develop cardiac failure resulting from destruction of a valve by infection. other indications to consider surgery include:

- unstable prosthetic valve or obstruction
- recurrent septic emboli, mycotic aneurysm
- large vegetations
- abscess formation
- early closure of mitral valve
- gram negative species

Infective endocarditis is associated with 25% mortality.

3. Non-infective endocarditis

Nonbacterial thrombic endocarditis (NBTE) or marantic endocarditis is most commonly found on previously undamaged valves.

As opposed to infective endocarditis, the vegetations in NBTE are small, sterile, and tend to aggregate along the edges of the valve or the cusps.

Also unlike infective endocarditis, NBTE does not cause an inflammation response from the body (confusing, as the suffix "-itis" refers to inflammation).

NBTE usually occurs during a hypercoagulable state such as system wide bacterial infection, or pregnancy, though it is also sometimes seen in patients with venous catheters. NBTE may also occur in patients with cancers, particularly mucinous adenocarcinoma (where Trousseau syndrome can be encountered). Typically NBTE does not cause many problems on its own, but parts of the vegetations may break off and embolize to the heart or brain, or they may serve as a focus where bacteria can lodge, thus causing infective endocarditis.

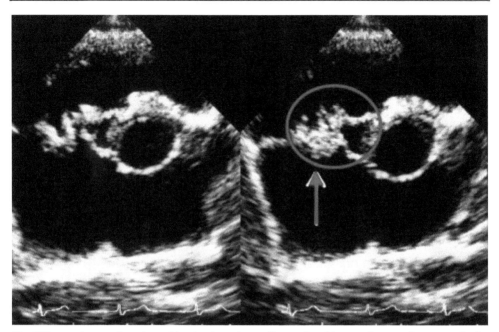

Fig. 2.Vegetation on the tricuspid valve by echocardiography. (Arrow denotes the vegetation)

Another form of sterile endocarditis, is termed LibmanSacks endocarditis; this form occurs more often in patients with lupus erythematosus and is thought to be due to the deposition of immune complexes. Like NBTE, LibmanSacks endocarditis involves small vegetations, while infective endocarditis is composed of large vegetations. These immune complexes precipitate an inflammation reaction, which helps to differentiate it from NBTE. Also unlike NBTE, LibmanSacks endocarditis does not seem to have a preferred location of deposition and may form on the under surfaces of the valves or even on the endocardium.] Prognosis:

Features suggestive of a worse prognosis are Acute endocarditis (Staphylococcus aureus), heart failure, IV drug abuse (often left and right sided disease), prosthetic valve infection, infection of the aortic rather than mitral valve, associated rhythm disturbance.

Subacute bacterial endocarditis (Streptococcus viridans) has a better prognosis.

4. References

[1] Mitchell RS, Kumar V, Robbins SL, Abbas AK, Fausto N (2007). *Robbins Basic Pathology* (8th ed.). Saunders/Elsevier. pp. 406–8.
[2] Morris AM (January 2006). "How best to deal with endocarditis". *Curr Infect Dis Rep* 8 (1): 14–22.
[3] Kasper DL, Brunwald E, Fauci AS, Hauser S, Longo DL, Jameson JL (May 2005). Harrison's Principles of Internal Medicine. McGraw-Hill. Pp
[4] Amal Mattu; Deepi Goyal; Barrett, Jeffrey W.; Joshua Broder; DeAngelis, Michael; Peter Deblieux; Gus M. Garmel; Richard Harrigan; David Karras; Anita L'Italien; David

Manthey (2007). Emergency medicine: avoiding the pitfalls and improving the outcomes. Malden, Mass: Blackwell Pub./BMJ Books. pp. 63.

[5] Taubert KA, Gewitz M, et al. (October 2007). "Prevention of infective endocarditis: guidelines from the American Heart Association". *Circulation* 116(15): 1736–54.

[6] Findler M, Livne S, et al. (December 2008). "Dentists' knowledge and implementation of the 2007 American Heart Association guidelines for prevention of infective endocarditis". *Oral Surg Oral Med Oral Pathol Oral Radiol Endod* 106(6): e16-9.

[7] Elad S, Binenfeld-Alon E, Zadik Y, Aharoni M, Findler M. (March 2011). of acceptance of the 2007 American Heart Association Guidelines for the prevention of infective endocarditis: A pilot study "Survey of acceptance of the 2007 American Heart Association guidelines for the prevention of infective endocarditis: a pilot study". *Quintessence Int* 42 (3): 243–51.

[8] Gold, JS; Bayar, S, Salem, RR (2004 Jul). "Association of Streptococcus bovis bacteremia with colonic neoplasia and extracolonic malignancy". Archives of surgery (Chicago, Ill. : 1960) 139 (7): 760-5.

[9] Durack D, Lukes A, Bright D (1994). "New criteria for diagnosis of infective endocarditis: utilization of specific echocardiographic findings. Duke Endocarditis Service". *Am J Med* 96 (3): 200–9.

[10] Weisse A, Heller D, Schimenti R, Montgomery R, Kapila R (1993). "The febrile parenteral drug user: a prospective study in 121 patients". *Am J Med* 94 (3): 274–80.

[11] Samet J, Shevitz A, Fowle J, Singer D (1990). "Hospitalization decision in febrile intravenous drug users". *Am J Med* 89 (1): 53–7.

[12] Marantz P, Linzer M, Feiner C, Feinstein S, Kozin A, Friedland G (1987). "Inability to predict diagnosis in febrile intravenous drug abusers". *Ann Intern Med* 106 (6): 823–8.

[13] Leibovici L, Cohen O, Wysenbeek A (1990). "Occult bacterial infection in adults with unexplained fever. Validation of a diagnostic index". *Arch Intern Med* 150 (6): 1270–2.

[14] Mellors J, Horwitz R, Harvey M, Horwitz S (1987). "A simple index to identify occult bacterial infection in adults with acute unexplained fever". *Arch Intern Med* 147 (4): 666–71.

[15] Kaech C, Elzi L, Sendi P, et al. (2006). "Course and outcome of Staphylococcus aureus bacteraemia: a retrospective analysis of 308 episodes in a Swiss tertiary-care centre". *Clin Microbiol Infect* 12 (4): 345–52.

Pathogenesis of Endocarditis – Bacteraemia of Oral Origin

Inmaculada Tomás-Carmona[1] and M. Álvarez-Fernández[2]
[1]Santiago de Compostela University
[2]Xeral-Cíes Hospital (Vigo)
Spain

1. Introduction

Bacteraemia is defined as the presence of bacteria in the blood. A feature that is unique to the oral bacterial biofilm, particularly the subgingival plaque biofilm, is its close proximity to a highly vascularised milieu. Any disruption of the natural integrity between the biofilm and the subgingival epithelium, which is at most about 10 cell layers thick, could lead to a bacteraemic state (Parahitiyawa et al., 2009). For several decades, the haematogenous spread of bacteria from the oral cavity has been considered a decisive factor in the pathogenesis of 10% to 15% of cases of infective endocarditis (IE); certain dental procedures may therefore carry a significant risk (Carmona et al., 2002). However, this statement has come under question, its detractors argue that not all patients with heart valves infected by bacteria that typically colonize ecological niches of the oral cavity have undergone dental procedures. Furthermore, there is as yet little evidence of genetic similarity between bacteria isolated from the heart valves, the bloodstream, and the oral cavity of patients with IE (Pallasch, 2003; Seymour et al., 2000).

Apart from its possible role in the onset of episodes of IE, bacteraemia of oral origin has attracted particular interest in the past two decades due to its possible involvement in the progression of atherosclerosis and its consequent implication in the development of ischaemic disease; however, the mechanism of action has not yet been fully elucidated (Beck et al., 1996; DeStefano et al., 1993; Olsen, 2008). A number of recently published clinical studies have demonstrated an association between periodontal disease and cardiovascular disease (Dietrich et al., 2008; Monteiro et al., 2009; Stein et al., 2009), and oral bacteria have been detected in atherosclerotic plaques, heart valves and aortic aneurysms (Gaetti-Jardim et al., 2009; Nakano et al., 2009; Pucar et al., 2007).

This chapter first provides a historical perspective of IE of oral origin. The models of the onset of IE of oral origin and the diagnostic methods for the detection and identification of oral bacteraemia are then discussed. This is followed by a critical review of bacteraemia secondary to dental procedures, focusing on prevalence, duration, magnitude and bacterial diversity, also analyzing factors that could favour the onset of bacteraemia. For this purpose, dental procedures have been divided into surgical and non-surgical, as invasive procedures are more likely to carry a higher risk. As the periodontal space is considered to be the principal portal of entry of bacteria into the bloodstream (Fig. 1), an independent analysis is performed of the dental procedures involving this anatomical region (periodontal procedures). Several authors have demonstrated that certain activities of daily living, such as chewing or toothbrushing, can also cause bacteraemia of oral origin; the importance of this observation is that these activities can significantly increase the number of episodes of bacteraemia compared to those produced exclusively by dental treatments. It has thus appeared appropriate to include a section on bacteraemia after everyday oral activities, including the concept known as "cumulative exposure", which encompasses this interesting aspect of bacteraemia of oral origin. The chapter concludes with a discussion of how current scientific evidence in the field of oral bacteraemia has influenced clinical practice guidelines on prophylaxis for IE of oral origin.

2. Historical perspective on infective endocarditis of oral origin

A focal infection is "a localised or generalised infection caused by the dissemination of microorganisms or toxic products from a focus of infection" (Easlick, 1951). The idea that many systemic infections could originate from infections of the oral cavity and that conservative dental treatment could favour this process took on special importance at the beginning of the 20th century. In 1900, William Hunter wrote: "Gold fillings, crowns and bridges built on and about diseased tooth roots form a veritable mausoleum over a mass of sepsis to which there is no parallel in the whole realm of medicine or surgery…" (Hunter, 1900).

Frank Billings was a key person in elaborating the concept and later dissemination of the theory of focal infection (Billings, 1916). He suggested that there was a possible relationship between the focus of infection, positive blood cultures and cardiac disease (Billings, 1909). Furthermore, this theory explained the origin of many acute systemic diseases and of a number of chronic diseases such as arthritis and nephritis (Billings, 1912). The microbiologist Edward Rosenow was Billings' most outstanding pupil, and his experiments on animal models permitted new theories to be elaborated which supported the importance of focal infection, including "bacterial transmutation" and "elective localisation" (Rosenow, 1914).

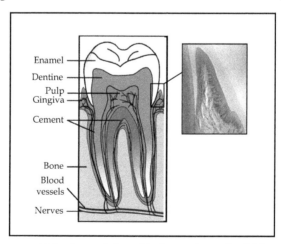

Fig. 1. Dental anatomy and histology of the critical area through which oral bacteria enter the bloodstream

After a period of popularity of the theory of focal infection, leading to the application of so-called "therapeutic edentulism" to many patients, the first detractors to this theory appeared in the 1930s (Holman, 1928). Reimann & Havens strenuously criticised Rosenow's experiments on the basis that, in many cases, the infectious agents had not been identified and that the patient's systemic disease did not reliably improve after dental extraction or tonsillectomy (Reimann & Havens, 1940).

However, in the forties and fifties there was a resurgence of the theory of focal infection, based mainly on the appearance in the medical literature of many cases of IE of oral origin (Bernstein, 1932; Brown, 1932; Geiger, 1942) and on epidemiological studies which revealed that the practice of dental extractions represented an important cause of IE (Kelson & White, 1945; Northrop & Crowley, 1943).

Okell & Elliott were the first authors to report bacteraemia after performing dental extractions; in a study of 138 patients undergoing such procedures, they detected bacteraemia due to *Streptococcus* species in 64% of cases (Okell & Elliott, 1935). A year later, Burket & Burn inoculated pigmented *Serratia marcescens* into the gingival sulcus of 90 patients before performing a dental extraction, isolating this bacterium in 20% of post-manipulation blood cultures. These results confirmed that microorganisms from the oral cavity could enter the bloodstream when performing a dental extraction (Burket & Burn, 1937). Between the mid 1930s and early 1950s numerous studies were published on the prevalence of post-extraction bacteraemia, reporting frequencies between 2% and 83% (Bender & Pressman, 1945; Hopkins, 1939; Palmer & Kempf, 1939; Rhoads et al., 1950; Robinson et al., 1950).

With respect to other oral activities, Richards performed a curious experiment in 1932 based on demonstrating whether "massage of a focus of infection" (located in joints, tonsils, gums, prostate or boils) caused the passage of bacteria into the bloodstream. In the case of the gums, the author selected 17 patients with gingivitis or the presence of periapical infection (confirmed by x-ray study) and massaged the gums or "moved" the teeth for 10 minutes; post-massage bacteraemia was detected in 3 cases (18%) (Richards, 1932) In 1941, Murray & Moosnick published an interesting study consisting of the extraction of blood cultures from patients with oral infections (active caries and/or periodontal disease) after chewing paraffin for 30 minutes. The blood cultures were positive for *Streptococcus* species in 185 (55%) of the 336 participants in this experiment (Murray & Moosnick, 1941).

In the early 1930s attention started to be paid to the need for IE prophylaxis in patients with valvular heart disease undergoing certain dental manipulations. Abrahamson & Brown, two of the pioneers of this idea, recommended the prophylactic use of autogenous vaccines (Abrahamson, 1931; Brown, 1932). In 1938, Feldman & Trace suggested cleaning and scraping the teeth prior to the manipulation in order to reduce contamination of the operating field, performing only 1 or 2 dental extractions per session, following the procedure with curettage and antiseptic irrigation of the periodontal pockets (Feldman & Trace, 1938). A year later, Elliott proposed perialveolar cauterization of the gingiva after dental extraction as a prophylactic measure, as this technique not only sterilized the sulcus but also sealed the gingival capillaries, thus preventing the passage of microorganisms into the bloodstream (Elliott, 1939). The practice of dental extractions under local infiltration anaesthesia with epinephrine was also recommended, as some authors had shown that this type of anaesthesia and this mode of administration acted as a barrier, preventing vascular invasion by the bacterial inoculum (Burket & Burn, 1937; Feldman & Trace, 1938). Fish &

Maclean recommended that the teeth of patients with IE be filled with cotton-wool soaked in a paste of zinc oxide and oil of cloves and that this was renewed every few days; those authors also recommended the administration of a dose of "prontosil" (azosulfamide) prior to dental extraction, in addition to cauterization of the gingiva (Fish & Maclean, 1936).

The first guidelines for antibiotic prophylaxis for IE associated with dental manipulations in patients with valvular heart disease were soon developed, and were based on the use of different sulfonamides (Hupp, 1993; Thomas et al., 1941). In 1948, Hirsh et al. were the first authors to investigate the effect of penicillin on the prevalence of post-extraction bacteraemia. The study group was composed of 65 control patients and 65 study patients, the latter group receiving 600,000 IU of penicillin intramuscularly 3 to 4 hours before the dental extraction; blood samples were taken immediately after the completion of surgery and at 10 and 30 minutes. Although the overall percentage of bacteraemia did not decline significantly (46% in controls *versus* 37% in those who received penicillin), the prevalence of streptococcal species in the positive blood cultures was significantly lower in patients who received prophylaxis compared with controls (15% *versus* 34%), confirming that penicillin was effective in reducing the prevalence of streptococcal bacteraemia, although not bacteraemia caused by other microorganisms (Hirsh et al., 1948).

In 1955, the American Heart Association (AHA), which at that time was formed by only seven physicians, developed its first protocol for IE prophylaxis before dental procedures. That protocol was recommended in patients with congenital or rheumatic heart disease who were undergoing dental extractions or other manipulations affecting the gingival tissues. Those experts considered that the fundamental principle of prophylaxis was to make high concentrations of antibiotic available in the bloodstream at the time of the manipulation and to maintain those levels for several days in order to eliminate the bacteria that had adhered to the heart valves during the bacteraemic episode. Their method of choice was based on the intramuscular injection of aqueous penicillin, 600,000 IU, and procaine penicillin, 600,000 IU, dissolved in oil with 2% aluminum monostearate and administered 30 minutes before the dental procedure. Alternatively (although less desirable), they proposed the oral administration of 250,000 IU to 500,000 IU of penicillin 30 minutes before each meal and before bedtime, starting 24 hours before the dental treatment and continuing for five days, with the administration of an extra dose of 250,000 IU of penicillin immediately before the procedure. For patients with a history of allergy to penicillin, the AHA recommended the use of other antibiotics such as oxytetracycline, chlortetracycline or erythromycin for five days starting the day before dental treatment (American Heart Association [AHA], 1955).

Later, several international committees, made up mainly of cardiologists, specialists in infectious diseases and pharmacologists, drew up alternative prophylactic regimens for IE in the context of dental procedures, describing the profile of the "susceptible patient" and the "at-risk" dental procedures. Those protocols have generated controversy and a degree of confusion.

3. Models of the development of infective endocarditis of oral origin

The classical model of the development of IE of oral origin is that the lesions occur in areas of damaged valvular endothelium, with accumulation of fibrin and platelet deposits constituting a so-called nonbacterial thrombotic endocarditis. This vegetation is sterile until invaded by oral microorganisms as a consequence of bacteraemia, with the subsequent onset of IE (Drangsholt, 1998) (Fig. 2).

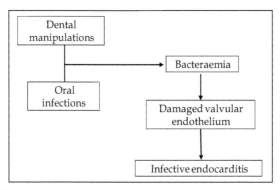

Fig. 2. Classical model of the development of infective endocarditis of oral origin

Several authors have demonstrated that bacteraemia of oral origin can play a significant role in the onset of atherosclerosis (Beck et al., 1996; DeStefano et al., 1993) and, based on these considerations, Drangsholt suggested that bacteraemia of oral origin, instead of directly inducing the onset of IE, could favour the initial thickening of the cardiac valves due to atherosclerosis, making them more susceptible to bacterial adherence and subsequent colonisation. He therefore proposed a new model for the pathogenesis of IE of oral origin, in which initially several episodes of bacteraemia would affect the endothelial surface of the cardiac valves over a long period of time, until finally a bacteraemic episode with a duration of days or weeks led to bacterial adherence and colonisation of the affected valve, culminating in an established cardiac infection (Drangsholt, 1998) (Fig. 3).

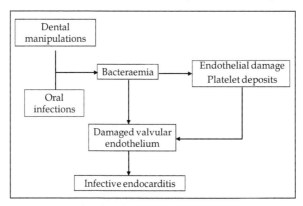

Fig. 3. A more recent model for the development of infective endocarditis of oral origin

Rather than an acute infectious disorder, this model describes IE of oral origin as a chronic disease with a long latency period and a number of well-defined stages. However, there is little evidence to support this model and few studies have been performed in experimental animals on the long-term effect of low-intensity bacteraemia of oral origin on the endothelial surface of the heart valves (Cohen et al., 2004).

4. Diagnostic methods for the detection and identification of bacteraemia of oral origin

There are several procedures for the microbiological analysis of blood cultures taken after dental procedures (Loza Fernández de Bobadilla et al., 2003; Romero et al., 1993). Early studies used quantitative methods that enabled the number of bacteria per millilitre of blood cultured to be determined; this technique was based on extending the blood sample on nutrient agar and then incubating (Elliott & Dunbar, 1968). However, it is recognized that this method is complex and requires expert staff, that it must be done at the time bacteraemia is suspected and the blood drawn and that it is not effective for the isolation of anaerobic bacteria (Romero et al., 1993).

In more recent papers on bacteraemia of oral origin, other authors used a lysis-centrifugation technique (Heimdahl et al., 1990), which is based on the collection and centrifugation of blood in a "Vacutainer system" tube with saponins that break down blood cells, followed by cultivation of the resulting pellet directly on the culture plates (Loza Fernández de Bobadilla et al., 2003; Romero et al., 1993). A variant of this technique is called lysis-filtration, in which, after the initial lysis stage, the blood is filtered and it is the filters that are cultivated directly on the culture plates (Hall et al., 1993). These two techniques enable semi-quantitative estimation to be performed by counting the colonies isolated, although it has been suggested that manipulation of the sample could increase the possibility of contamination (Loza Fernández de Bobadilla et al., 2003; Romero et al., 1993).

Qualitative methods have been used in many studies. In this method, blood is cultured in bottles with liquid or biphasic media (Roberts et al., 1997; Roberts et al., 1998b; Tomás et al., 2007). The culture medium must be examined each day to detect signs of bacterial growth. Although the conventional method involves daily visual inspection of the bottles, automated reading systems now exist based on the detection of the CO_2 produced by bacterial growth using radiometric or fluorimetric techniques, infrared spectroscopy, changes in pH, etc. (Loza Fernández de Bobadilla et al., 2003; Romero et al., 1993).

In 2002, Lucas et al. compared two techniques, lysis-filtration and the BACTEC system, for the analysis of post-dental extraction blood cultures in children. The results revealed that the BACTEC system is a quicker and more efficient method for the detection of both aerobic and anaerobic bacteria, particularly *Staphylococcus* spp. and some species of *Streptococcus,* and that it is able to detect extremely low levels of bacteraemia (Lucas et al., 2002a). Although the lysis-filtration technique allows the intensity of bacteraemia to be estimated, it requires immediate processing, whereas processing with the BACTEC system may be delayed up to 48 hours without affecting the bacterial detection rate (Chapin & Lauderdale, 1996). Nevertheless, after reviewing the literature on bacteraemia of oral origin, significant differences were detected between studies in relation not only to the microbiological technique applied, but also to the transport and culture media, atmosphere and incubation times used, as well as the characteristics of the phenotypic identification of the isolates (Diz et al., 2011; Tomás et al., 2011). All these factors could affect bacterial isolation and identification, particularly of fastidious oral bacteria. Some authors have therefore stated that "it is likely that oral bacteria recovered from blood by culture are probably only part of those present there" (Olsen, 2008). As a result, recently developed methods for the specific detection and identification of microorganisms, particularly polymerase chain reaction

(PCR) techniques, have brought renewed interest to this field, as shown by the studies performed by a number of authors (Kinane et al., 2005; Lockhart et al., 2008; Roberts et al., 2006; Savarrio et al., 2005; Sonbol et al., 2009).

In 2005, Savarrio et al., studying blood cultures taken during root canal treatment, found a lower prevalence of bacteraemia when using PCR analysis than they detected using conventional culture techniques (17% *versus* 30%) (Savarrio et al., 2005). However, Kinane et al., comparing conventional culture methods and PCR analysis, detected the following prevalences of bacteraemia: after ultrasonic scaling (13% by conventional culture and 23% by PCR), periodontal probing (20% and 16%, respectively) and toothbrushing (3% and 13%, respectively) (Kinane et al., 2005). Recently, Castillo et al. assessed the presence of subgingival pathogens (*Porphyromonas gingivalis, Aggregatibacter actinomycetemcomitans, Tannerella forsythia, Eikenella corrodens, Campylobacter rectus* and *Prevotella intermedia*) in peripheral blood samples from patients with periodontitis before and after scaling and root planing; their analysis was based on anaerobic culture and nested PCR. Specific bacterial DNA was detected in 14% of patients before the therapeutic intervention and in 19% after scaling and root planing. Although blood culture rendered higher detection rates immediately after the periodontal intervention, the prevalence fell significantly at subsequent sampling times, whereas detection by nested PCR was more uniform over the sampling period. Those authors therefore concluded that the use of these molecular-based techniques may improve the accuracy of results obtained by blood culture (Castillo et al., 2011).

In 2008, Bahrani-Mougeot et al. compared two different methods for the identification of oral bacteria from blood samples after dental extractions: biochemical analysis and sequence analysis of the 16S ribosomal RNA gene. Of the 58 bacteria isolated in their series, only 17% were identified as the same species by both methods, 55% belonged to the same genus but different species and 28% showed no correlation at all. Those authors stated that DNA sequencing resulted in more accurate identification of a more diverse population of bacteria in bacteraemia following dental extractions (Bahrani-Mougeot et al., 2008). On the other hand, the sensitivity of real-time, quantitative PCR techniques to quantify bacteraemia following dental manipulations has been limited up to now. In a paper published by Lockhart et al., the sensitivity of the method was 25 colony-forming units (CFU) per polymerase chain reaction, which corresponds to 10^3 to 10^4 CFU per millilitre of blood, all samples being below this detection threshold (Lockhart et al., 2008). Nevertheless, it has recently been demonstrated that real-time PCR with pyrosequencing can accurately identify microorganisms directly from positive blood culture bottles with the same sensitivity as culture-based methods (the two techniques were concordant for 97.8% of the bacteria) (Jordan et al., 2009).

The genetic relatedness between isolates from oral cavity and bloodstream samples may be analyzed by PCR techniques. Pérez-Chaparro et al., using a pulsed-field gel electrophoresis technique, recently confirmed the coexistence of the same bacterial clone in samples from the subgingival plaque and from peripheral blood in 16% of patients with bacteraemia following scaling and root planing (Pérez-Chaparro et al., 2008).

Hence, it is imperative that these molecular sequence-based approaches be validated and used in prospective trials to achieve a better understanding of the bacterial characteristics associated with oral bacteraemia.

5. Bacteraemia of oral origin

Numerous authors have studied the development of bacteraemia of oral origin, although the differences detected in the methodology used and in the characteristics of the study groups make it difficult to compare results from different series.

5.1 Baseline bacteraemia

A number of pioneers of the research into the field of bacteraemia of oral origin assumed that there was no bacteraemia at baseline (prior to any dental manipulation) and they therefore performed no pre-manipulation determinations in their studies (Giglio et al., 1992; Lockhart, 1996). However, in 2004, the British Society of Cardiology and the Royal College of Physicians of London were emphatic on this matter: "Those studies of bacteraemia of oral origin that do not to incorporate into their methodology a blood sample taken at baseline should not be considered evaluable" (British Society of Cardiology [BSC] & the Royal College of Physicians [RCP] of London, 2004).

Approximately 70% of the papers on bacteraemia following dental procedures include analysis of a baseline blood culture (Diz et al., 2011). In most of those studies the authors found that there was no bacteraemia rate before the intervention (Heimdahl et al., 1990; Okabe et al., 1995), although some authors reported positive blood cultures in 7% to 11% of cases (Roberts et al., 1998b; Savarrio et al., 2005). In 2005, Kinane et al., using PCR analysis, detected a baseline bacteraemia of 9% (Kinane et al., 2005). Roberts's group from the University of London deserves special mention; this group has repeatedly detected a higher prevalence of baseline bacteraemia in children (varying between 19% and 57%) (Lucas et al., 2002b; Lucas et al., 2007), although their results have not been confirmed by other authors studying paediatric patients. Surprisingly, Fine et al. recently detected a baseline bacteraemia (intensity of 1-2 CFU/ml) in half of adults with mild to moderate gingivitis (Fine et al., 2010). From a review of the literature, we have found that baseline bacteraemia is of very low intensity (median of the majority of series published to date, 0.33 CFU/ml). Although Lucas et al., in another paediatric case series, observed that baseline bacteraemia was mainly staphylococcal in nature (Lucas et al., 2002b; Lucas et al., 2007), Castillo et al., applying PCR analysis, recently detected *Prevotella gingivalis* in all patients with bacteraemia prior to scaling and root planing (Castillo et al., 2011).

To determine the prevalence of bacteraemia of oral origin it is essential to clarify its definition. Up to a few years ago, the detection of a positive post-dental manipulation blood culture was considered to indicate bacteraemia of oral origin. However, in 2004, the BSC and the RCP of London established a new concept of bacteraemia of oral origin defined as "that bacteraemia that is statistically significant with respect to the bacteraemia present at baseline" (BSC & RCP, 2004).

5.2 Bacteraemia following surgical and non-surgical procedures

5.2.1 Prevalence

In 1945, Bender & Pressman (Bender & Pressman, 1945) stated that the practice of dental extractions led to the entry of bacteria into the bloodstream due to the rupture of blood vessels in the gingival sulcus and the pumping effect induced by the manipulation. Over 70% of the literature on bacteraemia following oral surgery focuses on dental extraction as a procedure at risk of producing bacteraemia, probably because of the high frequency of this procedure and the associated bleeding (Diz et al., 2011).

An important aspect is the time at which the blood sample is collected. Roberts et al., in a study of 229 children undergoing dental extractions, determined the prevalence of bacteraemia at different times after completing the procedure (10, 60, 120, 180 and 600 seconds). They demonstrated that the optimum time for drawing the blood sample was 30 seconds after completion of the dental manipulation (Roberts et al., 1992). However, the time of collection of the post-manipulation blood sample varies between studies, ranging from "during" the procedure to 5 minutes after the completing treatment (Baltch et al., 1982; Josefsson et al., 1985; Okabe et al., 1995).

SURGICAL PROCEDURES	PREVALENCE OF BACTERAEMIA Median[1] (range)
Dental extractions	Children: 52% (30%-76%) Adults: 76% (58%-100%)
Extraction of third molars	49% (10%-62%)
Maxillofacial surgical techniques	18% (0%-58%)
Removal of osteosynthesis plates	8% (0%-20%)
Incision and drainage of abscesses	12%[‡]
Removal of oral sutures	10% (5%-16%)
Placement of dental implants	7%[2]
NON-SURGICAL PROCEDURES	PREVALENCE OF BACTERAEMIA Median[1] (range)
Conservative procedures	22% (4%-66%)
Orthodontic procedures	22% (7%-57%)
Endodontic procedures	15% (0%-42%)
Local anaesthetic techniques	73% (16%-97%)

[1]Median of the majority of series published to date.
[2]The absence of a prevalence range is due to there being only one paper on this subject in the literature reviewed.

Table 1. Prevalence of bacteraemia following surgical and non-surgical dental manipulations

A review of the literature revealed a prevalence of positive post-extraction blood cultures that varied between 30% and 76% in children and between 58% and 100% in adults.

Surprisingly, these percentages are significantly higher than those obtained after the extraction of impacted or partially erupted third molars (10%-62%) and after more aggressive maxillofacial surgical techniques (0%-58%) (Diz et al., 2011). Recently, Piñeiro et al. showed that even implant placement via a mucoperiosteal flap does not carry a significant risk of producing bacteraemia compared with the baseline percentage (the prevalence was 6.7% at 30 seconds and 3.3% at 15 minutes *versus* 2% at baseline) (Piñeiro et al., 2010) (Table 1). A possible explanation for these results is that the periodontal space is not invaded in these other surgical procedures, a factor which would suggest that this space represents the critical region from which oral bacteria enter the bloodstream (Parahitiyawa et al., 2009).

When evaluating non-surgical dental interventions (Table 1), the prevalence of bacteraemia was similar after conservative dental procedures (4%-66%) and after other orthodontic procedures (7%-57%), and was lower after performing root canal treatment (0%-42%) (Diz et al., 2011). In 1997, Roberts et al. were the first authors to study the prevalence of bacteraemia secondary to 13 different dental manipulations in 735 children undergoing dental treatment under general anaesthesia. Those authors found that matrix band insertion with a wooden wedge and the placement of a rubber dam led to a significant increase in the percentage of positive blood cultures compared to baseline conditions (32% and 29% *versus* 9%). However, low- and high-speed drilling led to positive blood cultures in a very small percentage of cases (4% and 13%, respectively) (Roberts et al., 1997). These findings were corroborated in subsequent studies conducted by the same research group (Roberts et al., 2000). According to Roberts et al., placement of a matrix band with a wooden wedge or placement of a rubber dam produces to changes in local pressures which could facilitate the passage of bacteria from the dental plaque to the gingival tissues (Roberts et al., 1997). In contrast, high- or low-speed drilling did not lead to a high prevalence of post-manipulation bacteraemia, questioning the initial hypothesis that these manoeuvres could break up bacterial plaque into small fragments which could easily penetrate the gingival spaces (Roberts et al., 2000).

In 2002, Lucas et al. used the lysis-filtration technique to analyze bacteraemia after different orthodontic procedures in a series of 142 children. Contrary to previous results (Erverdi et al., 1999; McLaughlin et al., 1996), those authors showed that the manipulation which caused the highest percentage of positive blood cultures was band cementation (44%), followed by the placement of interproximal separators (36%), the taking of alginate impressions (31%) and, finally, changing the archwire (19%). Curiously, despite the high percentage of positive blood cultures detected, the prevalence was not significantly higher than the baseline bacteraemia, which varied between 23% and 36%, so the post-manipulation bacteraemic episodes in that series should theoretically be considered as non-significant bacteraemia (Lucas et al., 2002b).

One of the first studies on the prevalence of bacteraemia secondary to endodontic procedures was performed by Bender et al. in 1960. Those authors stated that manipulation of the root canal involved a small, confined operating field with a significantly lower number of capillaries and blood vessels than are exposed when performing dental extractions or periodontal techniques; in addition, the operating field is usually isolated, avoiding contact with the saliva. These characteristics of endodontic treatment could explain the low prevalence of post-manipulation bacteraemia detected in the different series (Bender et al., 1960).

Regarding methods of local anaesthetic infiltration, Roberts et al. investigated the prevalence of bacteraemia after infiltrative, intraligamental and modified intraligamental techniques in children. The results showed that all three of the anaesthetic techniques caused to the passage of bacteria into the bloodstream, though there was a higher risk of bacteraemia with intraligamental injection (97% of cases) than with the modified intraligamental (50%) or infiltrative techniques (16%) (Roberts et al., 1998a). It has been suggested that bacteria which colonise the surfaces of the teeth at the border of the gingival sulcus are dragged into the sulcus by the tip of the needle and from there enter the blood vessels due to the high pressures generated by the intraligamental anaesthetic technique (Roberts, 1999). On the other hand, Lockhart suggested that injection of a local anaesthetic containing epinephrine could restrict the passage of bacteria into the circulatory system by reducing local blood flow (Lockhart, 1996).

A review of the literature has shown that, except for dental extraction and intraligamental anaesthesia, there are no significant differences in the prevalence of bacteraemia when performing surgical or non-surgical procedures (Diz et al., 2011) thus confirming that visible bleeding is not predictive of bacteraemia secondary to dental manipulations (BSC & RCP, 2004; Roberts, 1999). According to Roberts et al., invasion of the bloodstream by the bacterial inoculum is probably a consequence of the creation of a negative pressure which would lead to an aspiration effect of the bacteria towards the interior of the blood vessels. This pressure would form part of an intermittent positive and negative pressure cycle occurring during any dentogingival manipulation, with the exception of local anaesthetic techniques (which only induce high positive pressures at the time of injection). Microscopic changes occur in the gingival capillaries due to these pressure changes, facilitating bacterial access (Roberts, 1999).

5.2.2 Duration

Using dental extraction as the reference surgical procedure (due to the lack of published data on other surgical manipulations), it has been found that the prevalence of bacteraemia was 39% to 80% in the first 15 minutes after the manipulation, 10% to 40% at 30 to 45 minutes and 5% to 28% at 1 hour (Diz et al., 2011). In a study published by Roberts et al., in 2006 conducted on a group of 500 children undergoing dental extractions, the authors observed that the risk of a positive blood culture after performing an extraction was no longer statistically significant after 15 minutes (Roberts et al., 2006). These findings confirm the premise established by the AHA in the 1960s, that "bacteraemias of oral origin are transient and usually last no more than 15 minutes after completion of the dental manipulation" (AHA, 1960). Under physiological conditions, these bacteria are transferred from the bloodstream into tissues and are rapidly cleared by the reticuloendothelial system.

With regard to the duration of bacteraemia caused by non-surgical dental interventions, the majority of studies evaluated this aspect in the context of endodontic procedures, detecting positive blood cultures in 0% to 17% of patients in the first 10 minutes and 13% at 45 minutes after completion of root canal treatment (Diz et al., 2011). On the basis of the literature reviewed, it appears that the duration of bacteraemia following surgical and non-surgical dental treatments is related to the nature of the procedure and is prolonged after a dental extraction.

5.2.3 Intensity and bacterial diversity

It has been stated that bacteraemia secondary to dental procedures is usually of low intensity and contrasts with the high bacterial load used to induce IE in experimental animals (between 10^6 and 10^7 CFU/ml) (Carmona et al., 2002). The magnitude of bacteraemia caused by a surgical dental procedure varies between 0 and 300 CFU/ml (median of the majority of series published to date, 1.7 CFU/ml). Paradoxically, after relatively non-aggressive manoeuvres, such as an intraligamental injection or placement of a rubber dam, some authors detected bacteraemias in the range 10^3-10^5 CFU/ml (Roberts et al., 1998b; Roberts et al., 2000). However, in general it has been demonstrated that non-surgical dental treatments provoke bacteraemias of very low intensity (median of the majority of series published to date, 0.5 CFU/ml). Accordingly, taking into account the magnitude of bacteraemia at baseline (median of the majority series published to date, 0.33 CFU/ml), many of these episodes should be considered as non-significant bacteraemia (Lucas et al., 2002b; Lucas et al., 2007; Roberts et al., 2000; Sonbol et al., 2009). Nevertheless, conventional microbiological cultures could be providing us with inaccurate information on the true magnitude of the bacteraemia; this aspect may be improved in a near future through the use of quantitative PCR techniques.

Analysis of the literature shows that the bacteria most frequently isolated from blood cultures obtained after surgical dental interventions in adults (mainly dental extractions) were obligate anaerobic bacteria (50%), *Streptococcus* spp. (30%) and *Staphylococcus* spp. (5%) (Diz et al., 2011); however, Lockhart et al., applying PCR techniques, recently detected a high percentage of streptococcal isolates responsible for post-extraction bacteraemia (Lockhart et al., 2008). No data are available from large series on non-surgical interventions (Diz et al., 2011). In children, there was a predominance of *Streptococcus* spp. (55%) in the positive blood cultures taken after both surgical and non-surgical dental procedures; these were followed in frequency by *Staphylococcus* spp. (15%) and, at a much lower frequency, obligate anaerobic bacteria (1%-7%) (Diz et al., 2011). In recent paediatric case series in which patients underwent dental extractions or conservative dental procedures and bacteraemia was evaluated using PCR techniques, the predominant bacterial species identified in the positive post-manipulation blood cultures was *Streptococcus* spp. (Roberts et al., 2006; Sonbol et al., 2009).

5.2.4 Contributing factors

Most of the studies published on bacteraemia following surgical (mainly dental extractions) and non-surgical dental manipulations evaluated the influence of different factors on the development of bacteraemia of oral origin.

A number of paediatric case series published in the 1970s reported a frequency of post-extraction bacteraemia of 30% (Speck et al., 1976), significantly lower than the figures reported for adults (Shanson et al., 1978). Some authors suggested that the differences were due primarily to the small volume of blood drawn from younger patients (Robinson et al., 1950). In the past decade, despite the increased sensitivity of blood culture techniques, the prevalence of post-extraction bacteraemia detected in children is still lower than that reported in adults (Heimdahl et al., 1990; Roberts et al., 1998b). In 2009, Lockhart et al., using a logistic regression model, found that the prevalence of bacteraemia following dental extractions increased significantly with age (Lockhart et al. 2009).

Very few authors have analysed the influence of gender on the prevalence of oral bacteraemia. Okabe et al. reported no statistically significant gender-related differences in the prevalence of bacteraemia following dental extractions (Okabe et al., 1995). However, Tomás et al. detected a significantly higher prevalence of post-extraction bacteraemia at 15 minutes in females (with a higher value also observed at one hour), though no significant differences were observed in the oral health status between females and males (Tomás et al., 2007). It has been suggested that gender could affect the prevalence of certain septic episodes, although a higher susceptibility of one or other gender continues to be a subject of debate (Eachempati et al., 1999; Offner et al., 1999). Many experiments performed in animals have demonstrated that the immune response to bacteraemia could differ between males and females (Yanke et al., 2000) due to the immune modulating properties of the sex hormones on certain cells of the immune system on which specific receptors for these hormones have been identified (Angele et al., 2000).

Many authors have investigated whether the aggressiveness of different dental procedures could affect the prevalence of bacteraemia, although the results have been inconclusive. Elliott & Durban and Peterson & Peacock observed that the extraction of primary teeth caused bacteraemia in a considerable percentage of cases (32% and 36%, respectively), although in both series this was lower than the rate detected after the extraction of permanent teeth (64% and 61%, respectively) (Elliott & Durban, 1968; Peterson & Peacock, 1976). However, these findings have not been confirmed in more recent studies (Onçag et al., 2006). In agreement with the results of previous studies (Bender et al., 1963; Robinson et al., 1950), Okabe et al. found that the frequency of positive blood cultures increased significantly with the number of teeth extracted (65% in cases of one to five extractions compared with 100% in patients with more than 15 extractions) (Okabe et al., 1995). Subsequently, Roberts et al. also detected a higher percentage of bacteraemia (>50%) in children after multiple extractions compared with a single extraction (39%) (Roberts et al., 1997). In contrast, Coulter et al., in a series in children, observed that the number of teeth extracted did not influence the prevalence or intensity of post-extraction bacteraemia (Coulter et al., 1990), and Heimdahl et al. and Lockhart detected bacteraemia in almost 100% of adults after performing a single dental extraction (Heimdahl et al., 1990; Lockhart, 1996). In the series published by Tomás et al., the number of teeth extracted did not influence the prevalence of bacteraemia at 30 seconds, 15 minutes or one hour post-extraction (Tomás et al., 2007)

Some authors demonstrated an association between the severity of haemorrhage secondary to the surgical manipulation and the appearance of bacteraemia (more than 90% of patients with a blood loss exceeding 50 ml developed bacteraemia compared to 67% when the blood loss was less than 10 ml) (Okabe et al., 1995). In contrast, Takai et al. found that the prevalence of bacteraemia associated with various oral and maxillofacial surgical procedures was not affected by blood loss during surgery (Takai et al., 2005). Okabe et al. studied the effect of the duration of surgery and found that when the operation exceeded 100 minutes the frequency of post-extraction bacteraemia was 96% compared to 67% when the surgery was of shorter duration (Okabe et al., 1995); however, other authors have reported conflicting results (Josefsson et al., 1985).

With respect to minor surgical manipulations, Giglio et al. observed that the risk of bacteraemia associated with the removal of sutures was directly related to the number of sutures removed, as positive blood cultures were only obtained from patients in whom five or more sutures were removed (Giglio et al., 1992).

In non-surgical dental procedures, Bender et al. demonstrated that although vitality of the pulp did not affect the prevalence of bacteraemia following endodontic procedures, the percentage of positive blood cultures varied with the depth of the instrumentation. When instrumentation was performed within the limits of the root canal, bacteria did not necessarily reach the general circulation, but with trans-apical instrumentation the bacteria were introduced directly into the interior of the vascular structures (Bender et al., 1960). Debelian et al., despite recognising the statistical limitations of the small size of their sample, reported no significant differences in the prevalence of post-endodontic bacteraemia according to the degree of periapical invasion or the size of the periapical lesion (Debelian et al., 1995).

Few studies have been published on the influence of the anaesthetic modality (local *versus* general anaesthesia) on the development of bacteraemia of oral origin, and the results are not consistent (Baltch et al., 1982; Keosian et al., 1956; Takai et al., 2005). In a paper published in 1956, a higher percentage of positive post-extraction blood cultures was detected after surgery under local anaesthesia than under general anaesthesia (26% *versus* 13%) (Keosian et al., 1956). In 2005, Takai et al. reported a similar prevalence of post-manipulation bacteraemia in patients undergoing extractions under general anaesthesia and under local anaesthesia (57.7% and 58.1%, respectively) (Takai et al., 2005). In contrast, Barbosa et al. found that the prevalence and duration of bacteraemia following dental extractions was higher in patients treated under general anaesthesia than in those treated under local anaesthesia (at 30 seconds, 89% *versus* 53%; at 15 minutes, 64% *versus* 24%; and at one hour, 21% *versus* 4%), suggesting that the practice of dental treatment under general anaesthesia could be a risk factor for bacteraemia. Those authors considered three hypotheses associated with general anaesthesia to explain the results obtained in their series: the appearance of bacteraemia secondary to the manoeuvres of nasotracheal intubation, the transitory changes in blood flow and in the immune response caused by the anaesthetic agents, and other factors such as the administration of contaminated anaesthetic agents (Barbosa et al., 2010).

With regard to oral health status, it appears that the number of teeth present in the mouth, their state of decay, and the existence of periapical abscesses do not alter the risk of post-intervention bacteraemia (Brennan et al., 2007; Coulter et al., 1990; Roberts et al., 1998b; Takai et al., 2005; Tomás et al., 2007). Some paediatric case series have reported significant differences in gingival inflammation scores between children with post-extraction bacteraemia and those with negative blood cultures (Roberts et al., 1998b). In addition, Roberts et al. suggested that the health of gingival tissues not only conditioned the prevalence of post-extraction bacteraemia but also probably its intensity by influencing the size of the bacterial inoculum (Roberts et al., 1998b). However, the majority of the authors consider that the state of gingival and periodontal health is not a determining factor in either surgical or non-surgical interventions (Burden et al., 2004; Lockhart et al., 2009; Lucas et al., 2002b; Roberts et al., 2000; Takai et al., 2005; Tomás et al., 2007), although it has been observed that the prevalence of post-extraction bacteraemia increased in the presence of an acute infectious process affecting the teeth (Okabe et al., 1995; Takai et al., 2005). For example, Takai et al. reported a significant increase in the prevalence of bacteraemia after the extraction of teeth with some type of infection (periodontal or periapical infection or pericoronitis) compared to the prevalence detected after the extraction of uninfected teeth (68% *versus* 23%) (Takai et al., 2005).

5.3 Bacteremia following periodontal procedures

5.3.1 Prevalence

The special interest of periodontal procedures is that they involve manipulation of the critical area through which oral bacteria enter the bloodstream (Fig. 1). Table 2 shows the prevalence of bacteraemia after different periodontal procedures.

The literature shows that surgical periodontal treatments (the most invasive procedures in terms of aggressiveness due to the need for dissection of a mucoperiosteal flap) are associated with a prevalence of bacteraemia of 39% to 60%. Approximately half of the published articles on bacteraemia following periodontal procedures focus on scaling as a procedure at risk of producing bacteraemia, with a reported prevalence that ranged from 8% to 77%. Similar figures have been reported after dental cleaning procedures (15%-60%). Less invasive manoeuvres, such as subgingival irrigation or periodontal probing (which is the introduction of a probe into the periodontal space for diagnostic purposes), can provoke bacteraemia in 0% to 30% and 10% to 40% of cases, respectively (Diz et al., 2011).

In 1973, Lineberger & De Marco studied the prevalence of bacteraemia associated with different periodontal manipulations (gingivectomy, flap surgery and/or osteoplasty) in 20 patients with chronic periodontitis, differentiating between those who had undergone previous periodontal treatment (scaling and routine dental prophylaxis) and those who had not. Although the size of the sample means that the results must be viewed with caution, they detected positive post-periodontal-surgery blood cultures in 50% of patients (Lineberger & De Marco, 1973). In studies in children undergoing dental treatment under general anaesthesia, Roberts et al. found that, after raising a mucoperiosteal flap, bacteraemia was detected in 39% to 43% of cases (Roberts et al., 1997; Roberts et al., 1998b).

Witzenberger et al. observed that 55% of patients with periodontitis developed bacteraemia after scaling and root planing (Witzenberger et al., 1982). Recently Lafaurie et al. and Maestre et al., in studies of adult patients with periodontitis, detected bacteria in the blood in 74% and 76%, respectively, of patients immediately after scaling and root planing (Lafaurie et al., 2007; Maestre et al., 2008). Other authors have shown that almost 30% of children develop bacteraemia secondary to professional cleaning with a rubber cup (De Leo et al., 1974; Roberts et al., 1997). Lucas & Roberts, in a paediatric case series, compared the prevalence of bacteraemia after scaling and after rubber-cup cleaning, finding no statistically significant difference in the number of positive blood samples in the groups studied (40% and 25%, respectively) (Lucas & Roberts, 2000).

In 1997 the AHA advised against the application of antiseptics using gingival irrigators (Dajani et al., 1997), probably assuming that the practice of subgingival irrigation could favour the passage of oral bacteria into the bloodstream. However, few papers have been published on this subject and their results are contradictory. Witzenberger et al. and Lofthus et al. studied bacteraemia secondary to subgingival irrigation in patients with periodontal pockets with a depth equal to or greater than 4 mm and macroscopic bleeding. Witzenberger et al. did not detect any positive post-manipulation blood cultures whereas

Lofthus et al. reported a bacteraemia rate of 30% (6 of 20 patients) at 2 minutes after irrigation (Lofthus et al., 1991; Witzenberger et al., 1982). Daly et al. observed bacteraemia after periodontal probing in 43% of subjects with untreated periodontal disease (Daly et al., 1997), while Kinane et al. recently detected positive post-probing blood cultures in 18% of volunteers with untreated periodontal disease, a prevalence similar to that detected by the same authors after ultrasonic scaling. Those authors suggested that detectable bacteraemia induced by periodontal procedures may be less intense than previously reported. Adult patients with periodontitis could represent a unique patient base whose immune systems are highly primed to cope with periodontal bacteria, such that when bacteraemia is induced it is quickly and efficiently cleared by the patient's reticuloendothelial system (Kinane et al., 2005). Roberts et al. performed a dental examination based on the removal of bacterial plaque close to the gingival margin (without performing probing of the sulcus) in 53 children, detecting positive post-manipulation blood cultures in 17% of cases (Roberts et al., 1997).

In the literature reviewed, there were no significant differences in the prevalence of bacteraemia when performing surgical or non-surgical (mainly scaling and dental cleaning procedures) periodontal interventions; this would indicate that visible bleeding is not a predictive factor for bacteraemia secondary to dental manipulations (Roberts, 1999).

PERIODONTAL PROCEDURES	PREVALENCE OF BACTERAEMIA Median[1] (range)
Periodontal surgery	42% (39%-60%)
Scaling	40% (8%-77%)
Professional cleaning	27% (15%-60%)
Subgingival irrigation	15% (0%-30%)[2]
Periodontal probing	18% (10%-40%)

[1]Median of the majority of series published to date.
[2]Mean has been expressed due to the small number of series published to date

Table 2. Prevalence of bacteraemia following different periodontal procedures

5.3.2 Duration

There are very few references in the literature that have evaluated the duration of bacteraemia following periodontal treatment. In early series, bacteraemic episodes persisted for at least 30 minutes in more than a third of patients undergoing ultrasound scaling (Baltch et al., 1982). Recently, Forner et al. detected bacteraemia in 13% of patients at 10 minutes after performing scaling and in 5% at 30 minutes (Forner et al., 2006). In contrast, Lafaurie et al., after performing scaling and root planing, detected positive blood cultures in 38% at 15 minutes and in 19% at 30 minutes after completion of the periodontal manipulation (Lafaurie et al., 2007).

5.3.3 Intensity and bacterial diversity

Although the authors of some studies in adults have reported that the bacteria most frequently isolated were *Streptococcus* spp., followed by obligate anaerobic bacteria (Daly et al., 1997; Forner et al., 2006), other authors have identified a predominance of obligate anaerobic bacteria in post-scaling bacteraemia, particularly periodontopathogenic bacteria such as *Porphyromonas gingivalis, Micromonas micros, Aggregatibacter actinomycetemcomitans, Prevotella* spp. and *Fusobacterium nucleatum* (Castillo et al., 2011; Lafaurie et al., 2007; Maestre et al., 2008). In a study of children undergoing various periodontal manipulations, the bacteria identified in positive post-manipulation blood cultures were mainly streptococci and staphylococci (Lucas & Roberts, 2000).

5.3.4 Contributing factors

The studies reviewed on bacteraemia following periodontal procedures showed considerable heterogeneity in methodological issues such as periodontal diagnosis, and the small sample size in some of the studies may have affected the statistical significance of the results obtained. Lineberger & De Marco determined the prevalence of bacteraemia associated with different periodontal surgical manipulations in patients with chronic periodontitis, observing no influence of age or sex on the results (Linerberger & De Marco, 1973). Equally, in other series, it has been demonstrated that the magnitude of post-scaling bacteraemia was not affected by age, gender, smoking or the duration of scaling (Forner et al., 2008).

Forner et al. showed that the prevalence and magnitude of bacteraemia after scaling was significantly higher in patients with periodontitis than in patients with gingivitis or healthy controls (Forner et al., 2008). Daly et al. studied the prevalence of positive blood cultures after periodontal probing in adults with untreated periodontitis and compared the results with those obtained in patients with chronic gingivitis. Patients with periodontal disease presented nearly a six-fold increase in the risk of developing bacteraemia compared with patients with gingivitis (Daly et al., 2001). Other authors, however, found no statistical differences in the prevalence or magnitude of post-scaling bacteraemia between patients with chronic periodontitis and those with aggressive periodontitis (Forner et al., 2008; Lafaurie et al., 2007). In children, the percentages of bacteraemia following scaling and rubber-cup cleaning were not affected by the plaque or gingival indices. Nevertheless, it seems that the presence of periodontal disease does condition the development of bacteraemia when performing periodontal treatment.

With regard to the influence of other factors, Reinhardt et al. showed that the use of sterile water *versus* non-sterile water during scaling with ultrasound did not affect the prevalence or intensity of post-manipulation bacteraemia (Reinhardt et al., 1982). Lofthus et al. detected no significant differences in the prevalence of post-irrigation bacteraemia when chlorhexidine or sterile water was used as the irrigating solution (Lofthus et al., 1991).

5.4 Bacteraemia following everyday oral activities

5.4.1 Prevalence

Everyday oral activities such as toothbrushing, dental flossing, use of water irrigation devices or chewing can provoke bacteraemia, possibly because these activities produce small movements of the tooth within the socket, causing intermittent positive and negative pressures that favour the movement of microorganisms into the bloodstream (Roberts, 1999). Specifically, it is estimated that the prevalence of bacteraemia attributable to toothbrushing is of 0% to 62% (median of the majority of series published to date, 22%), the risk with the use of irrigation devices is of 0% to 50% (median of the majority of series published to date, 13%) and the lowest risk is with chewing (median of the majority of series published to date, 3%) (Table 3) (Diz et al., 2011).

EVERYDAY ORAL ACTIVITIES	PREVALENCE OF BACTERAEMIA Median[1] (range)
Toothbrushing	22% (0%-62%)
Supragingival irrigation	13% (0%-50%)
Flossing	19% (0%-41%)
Chewing	3% (0%-17%)

[1]Median of the majority of series published to date.

Table 3. Prevalence of bacteraemia following everyday oral activities

Studies on bacteraemia following everyday oral activities in both adults and children have focused principally on bacteraemia after toothbrushing (Diz et al., 2011). Madsen demonstrated that both toothbrushing and the use of toothpicks produced bacteraemia in 36% of patients with gingival and periodontal alterations (Madsen, 1974). Schlein et al. determined the percentage of positive blood cultures five minutes after completing toothbrushing and found that 25% of subjects had post-activity bacteraemia (Schlein et al., 1991). Roberts et al. and Lucas et al. demonstrated in various studies in children that almost 40% of subjects developed bacteraemia secondary to toothbrushing (Roberts et al., 1997; Lucas et al., 2008), while others authors detected prevalences of up to 62% (Bhanji et al., 2002). In contrast, in recent studies such as those published by Hartzell et al. and Jones et al., the rate of bacteraemia following toothbrushing was zero (Hartzell et al., 2005; Jones et al., 2010). However, it is important to note that the study group in the series published by Jones et al. was formed of mechanically ventilated adults, of whom 87% were receiving empirical antibiotic therapy, which could have affected the results (Jones et al., 2010).

Although some authors were unable to show that supragingival irrigation with water produced a bacteraemic episode (Romans & App, 1971; Tamimi et al, 1969), Felix et al. found that half of the patients with periodontitis who performed this procedure for one minute presented positive post-manipulation blood cultures (Felix et al., 1971). Berger et al. investigated the prevalence of bacteraemia secondary to the use of an oral irrigator for one minute in subjects with no gingival or periodontal disease and, of the 30 individuals evaluated, eight (27%) had positive blood cultures at one minute after completing the irrigation compared to none after simple toothbrushing (Berger et al., 1974). Ramadan et al. found that 18% of patients with advanced periodontitis yielded positive blood cultures after the use of dental floss or Stim-U-Dents, while Crasta et al. recently reported that 40% of subjects presented positive blood cultures after flossing (Crasta et al., 2009; Ramadan et al., 1975).

Although Cobe demonstrated in 1954 that chewing a hard sweet led to bacteraemia in 17% of patients (Cobe, 1954), Degling did not detect positive blood cultures in any patients with fixed orthodontic appliances after chewing gum for five minutes (Degling, 1972). Similarly, Murphy et al. recently showed that chewing did not cause bacteraemia in patients with chronic periodontitis or plaque-induced gingivitis and that this activity may not be a risk factor for IE (Murphy et al., 2006). Schlegel et al. performed an interesting experiment on dogs in which dental implants had been placed nine months earlier; those authors looked for the presence of bacteraemia after inoculating a suspension of *Staphylococcus aureus* into the peri-implant sulcus and allowing the animals to eat for five minutes. They did not detect any positive blood cultures. Together with the histological findings, this allowed the authors to suggest that the epithelium and connective tissue surrounding the implants acted as a barrier as if it were a "physiological pocket" (Schlegel et al., 1978).

Various authors have compared the prevalence of bacteraemia following everyday oral activities, mainly toothbrushing, with that detected after performing certain dental treatments (Forner et al., 2006; Kinane et al., 2005, Lockhart et al., 2008; Lucas & Roberts, 2000). Lineberger & De Marco analysed the frequency of bacteraemia secondary to the use of dental floss and of a gingival stimulator, finding that between 20% and 30% of patients had positive post-manipulation blood cultures, compared to 50% of patients undergoing periodontal surgery (Lineberger & De Marco, 1973). Lockhart et al. detected a significantly lower number of positive cultures in patients performing toothbrushing than in those undergoing dental extractions (19% and 58%, respectively) (Lockhart et al., 2008). Forner et al. studied the prevalence of positive blood cultures after toothbrushing, chewing and scaling, detecting a significantly lower percentage of bacteraemia after toothbrushing (1.6%) and chewing (6.6%) than after scaling (35%) (Forner et al., 2006). In the series by Kinane et al., the prevalences of bacteraemia after the different activities were the following: toothbrushing, 8%; periodontal probing, 18%; and ultrasonic scaling, 18% (Kinane et al., 2005). In contrast, Lucas & Roberts found no significant differences in the prevalence of positive blood cultures between three groups (toothbrushing, 39%; professional cleaning with a rubber cup, 25%; and scaling, 40%) (Lucas & Roberts, 2000).

5.4.2 Duration

Approximately one third of the publications on bacteraemia following everyday oral activities have evaluated the duration of bacteraemia. It has been found that the prevalence of bacteraemia was 0% to 20% in the first 15 minutes after the activity, 0% to 1% at 20 to 40 minutes and of 2% at one hour (Diz et al., 2011). It may therefore be said that bacteraemia following everyday oral activities does not usually persist for more than 15 minutes and that the duration is shorter than is observed after performing dental extractions.

5.4.3 Intensity and bacterial diversity

Bacteraemia following everyday oral activities is generally of low intensity (median of the series published to date, 0.97 CFU/ml; range; 0.01-32 CFU/ml), although its magnitude is significantly higher than the baseline bacteraemia observed in the same series (median of the series published to date, 0.02 CFU/ml; range, 0.01-0.05 CFU/ml). In the study by Forner et al., the intensity of bacteraemia following everyday oral activities (toothbrushing and chewing) was significantly lower than those authors detected after scaling (0.11 CFU/ml and 0.19 CFU/ml *versus* 0.78 CFU/ml) (Forner et al., 2006). In contrast, the results published by Lucas & Roberts revealed that the intensity of bacteraemia was higher after toothbrushing (32.2 ± 231 CFU/ml) than after professional cleaning with a rubber cup or scaling (15.9 ± 83.5 CFU/ml and 2.2 ± 13.2 CFU/ml, respectively) (Lucas & Roberts, 2000). Nevertheless, analysis of the intensity of bacteraemia following everyday oral activities must take into account the constraints of microbiological quantification techniques, given the indirect information provided by conventional culture and the limitations of sensitivity of quantitative-PCR when dealing with a very small bacterial inoculum (Lockhart et al., 2008).

In the literature reviewed, the most frequently isolated bacteria in positive post-toothbrushing blood cultures were *Streptococcus* spp. (45%) followed by obligate anaerobes (19%) and *Staphylococcus* spp. (15%). Lockhart et al., applying a 16S ribosomal RNA sequencing method for bacterial identification, observed that 48% of positive cultures in the toothbrushing group were viridans group streptococci (Lockhart et al., 2008).

5.4.4 Contributing factors

Toothbrushing is the activity of everyday living for which there is most evidence regarding the influence of different factors that may contribute to the prevalence of bacteraemia. Lockhart et al. demonstrated that older age was a predictive factor for developing bacteraemia after toothbrushing (Lockhart et al., 2009). There is also a widely held view that the probability of developing bacteraemia after toothbrushing using an electric toothbrush could be higher than after using a manual toothbrush (Bhanji et al., 2002; Misra et al., 2007).

Lockhart et al. found no significant relationship between the prevalence of bacteraemia after toothbrushing and any measures of caries (presence and depth of caries, presence and size of apical lucency) (Lockhart et al., 2009). In a number of papers on bacteraemia following toothbrushing, various authors found no statistically significant relationship between the state of oral hygiene or the gingival or periodontal status and the prevalence of bacteraemia (Hartzell et al., 2005; Kinane et al., 2005; Madsen, 1974; Schlein et al., 1991; Sconyers et al., 1973). However, in patients with moderate and high plaque indices (PI≥ 1.51) and gingival indices (GI≥ 1.51), Silver et al. detected a prevalence of bacteraemia of 60% and 62%, respectively, after toothbrushing compared to 35% and 25%, respectively, in patients with low PI and GI (scores of 0–1.50). Those authors also demonstrated that positive post-toothbrushing blood cultures with isolation of more than three different bacterial species were significantly more common in patients with a GI equal to or greater than 1.51 than in those with a GI of 0 to 1.50 (28% *versus* 2%)(Silver et al., 1977). Lockhart et al., analysing the influence of a number of clinical parameters, found that a PI equal to or greater than 2 (OR, 3.78), a calculus index (CI) equal to or greater than 2 (OR, 4.43) and the type of bleeding (generalised bleeding) after the activity (OR, 7.96) had a significant effect on the prevalence and duration of post-toothbrushing bacteraemia (Lockhart et al., 2009). One of the authors of the present chapter (Tomás et al., 2011) performed a meta-analysis in order to clarify the influence of oral hygiene and gingival and periodontal status on the development of bacteraemia from everyday oral activities. The results obtained in that meta-analysis showed a significant influence of the plaque and gingival indices (0-1.50 *versus* ≥ 1.51) on the prevalence of bacteraemia following toothbrushing.

With respect to other everyday oral activities, Murphy et al. stated that differing consistencies of the various chewing mediums might contribute to the differences in the reported prevalence of bacteraemia following chewing (Murphy et al., 2006). Cobe showed that chewing hard candy provoked a higher percentage of bacteraemia than did chewing gum (17.4% *versus* 0%) (Cobe, 1954). Few published studies have looked at the influence of oral hygiene and gingival and periodontal status on the prevalence of bacteraemia after performing dental flossing or chewing. In those studies, there was no statistically significant association between the state of oral hygiene or gingival or periodontal status and the prevalence of bacteraemia (Crasta et al., 2006; Fine et al., 2010; Forner et al., 2006; Murphy et al., 2006; Robinson et al., 1950).

5.5 "Cumulative exposure"

Although the potential clinical impact of these episodes of low-level bacteraemia caused by everyday oral activities is unknown, its significance is based on the so-called "cumulative exposure" (Guntheroth, 1984; Roberts, 1999). In 1984, Guntheroth estimated the cumulative exposure to bacteraemia over a period of one month after a tooth extraction and compared this to the results obtained after toothbrushing, during chewing and "in situations of oral sepsis". For this purpose, he multiplied the duration of bacteraemia, expressed in minutes per day, by its prevalence in each situation and calculated that in one month, the cumulative exposure to bacteraemia secondary to two extractions was of only six minutes, whereas this reached 120 minutes after toothbrushing, 510 minutes with chewing and 4,740 minutes with "physiological bacteraemia due to oral sepsis" (Guntheroth, 1984).

In 1999, Roberts repeated the estimation of cumulative exposure to bacteraemia applying a similar methodology to that used by Guntheroth but with certain modifications: to the frequency of positive post-dental-manipulation blood cultures and the duration of the episodes (assuming a mean time of 15 minutes), as applied by Guntheroth, he added the size of the bacterial inoculum and estimated the number of dentogingival procedures that a patient with cardiac pathology would undergo in a period of one year. Roberts calculated the index of cumulative exposure as an expression of the "relative risk" of developing bacteraemia after a certain dental procedure by comparing the results with those obtained after a standard manipulation (extraction of a deciduous molar). In that study, certain conservative dental procedures, such as the placement of a rubber dam, led to a risk of cumulative exposure to bacteraemia 2,110,341 times higher than the extraction of a deciduous molar, and toothbrushing (twice a day) carried a risk 154,219 times higher than the dental extraction. He also attributed a high risk of cumulative exposure to bacteraemia of oral origin to the activities of everyday living in patients with and without oral infection (7,691,707 and 5,640,585 times higher, respectively, than a deciduous tooth extraction) (Roberts, 1999).

Three years later, the Roberts' research group estimated the cumulative exposure to bacteraemia (expressed as the number of CFU/ml/min/year) secondary to various dental procedures in a group of 136 children with cardiac pathology, differentiating between dental manipulations in which the administration of antibiotic prophylaxis was indicated and those in which it was not. According to those authors, the placement of a rubber dam caused the highest value of cumulative exposure (8,849,000 CFU/ml/min/year) and the extraction of a deciduous tooth the lowest (0.059 CFU/ml/min/year). Dental examination produced a cumulative exposure of 1,999 CFU/ml/min/year and rubber-cup dental polishing with prophylactic paste an exposure of 16,410 CFU/ml/min/year (Al-Karaawi et al., 2001).

Despite the above, experts on this subject such as Delahaye & De Gevigney suggested that caution should be observed in the interpretation of this "theoretical analysis", as factors such as the duration of the bacteraemia could vary between patients. According to those authors, a prospective study must be designed in order to analyse all the components of cumulative exposure to bacteraemia individually. The concept of "cumulative exposure" has generated significant controversy in the scientific community (Delahaye & De Gevigney, 2001).

6. Current perspective on the prevention of infective endocarditis of oral origin

The American Heart Association (AHA) published the first protocol for the prevention of IE associated with dental procedures in 1955 (AHA, 1955). Since that time, many expert committees in different countries have drawn up distinct prophylactic regimens, many of which have subsequently been revised and modified based on different types of studies, including those on the prevalence of bacteraemia secondary to dental procedures.

In the latest guidelines published by the British Society for Antimicrobial Chemotherapy, the AHA, the National Institute for Health and Clinical Excellence (NICE) of the United Kingdom, and the European Society of Cardiology (Gould et al., 2006; Habib et al., 2009; Wilson et al., 2007; National Institute for Health and Clinical Excellence [NICE], 2008), the emphasis for the cause of IE has shifted from procedure-related bacteraemia to cumulative bacteraemia due to everyday oral activities. NICE considered that it was "biologically implausible" that a dental procedure could lead to a greater risk of IE than regular toothbrushing (NICE, 2008). Some of those expert committee guidelines concurred with the premise: "Maintenance of optimal oral hygiene and periodontal health may reduce the incidence of bacteraemia following everyday oral activities and is more important than prophylactic antibiotics for a dental procedure to reduce the risk of IE" (NICE, 2008; Wilson et al. 2007). NICE has adopted a drastic stance in this respect, issuing the statement that "antibiotic prophylaxis for IE is not recommended in individuals undergoing dental procedures" (NICE, 2008).

7. Conclusions

Apart from its possible implication in the onset of episodes of IE, there has been increasing interest in bacteraemia of oral origin in the past two decades due to the major role it is considered to play in the progression of atherosclerosis and consequently in the occurrence of chronic diseases.

It is imperative that molecular sequence-based approaches be validated and used in prospective trials to achieve a better understanding of the bacterial characteristics associated with bacteraemia of oral origin.

Dental extraction is the procedure that carries the highest risk of bacteraemia in terms of prevalence, duration and magnitude. There is no conclusive evidence on the contributing factors that predispose to the development of bacteraemia in patients undergoing dental procedures, although it is likely that gingival and periodontal health is relevant to the onset of bacteraemia when performing periodontal interventions.

Activities of everyday living, such as chewing and toothbrushing, can also cause bacteraemia and their clinical importance is based on the concept of "cumulative exposure to bacteraemia". A meta-analysis showed that elevated plaque accumulation and gingival inflammation scores significantly increase the prevalence of bacteraemia following toothbrushing.

Scientific evidence in the field of oral bacteraemia has greatly influenced clinical practice guidelines on prophylaxis against IE of oral origin.

8. Acknowledgement

This work was supported by Xunta de Galicia (Grant PGIDT 08CSA010208PR), Spain.

9. References

Abrahamson, L. (1931). Subacute bacterial endocarditis following removal of septic foci. *British Medical Journal*, Vol.2, No.3678, pp.8-9, ISSN 0007-1447.

Al-Karaawi, ZM., Lucas, VS., Gelbier, M., & Roberts, GJ. (2001). Dental procedures in children with severe congenital heart disease: a theoretical analysis of prophylaxis and non-prophylaxis procedures. *Heart*, Vol.85, No.1, pp.66-68, ISSN 1355-6037.

American Heart Association. (1955). Prevention of rheumatic fever and bacterial endocarditis through control of streptococcal infections. *Circulation*, Vol.11, pp.317-320, ISSN 0009-7322.

American Heart Association. (1960). Prevention of rheumatic fever and bacterial endocarditis through control of streptococcal infections. *Circulation*, Vol.21, pp.151-155, ISSN 0009-7322.

Angele, MK., Schwacha, MG., Ayala, A., & Chaudry, IH. (2000). Effect of gender and sex hormones on immune responses following shock. *Shock: Molecular, Cellular, and Systemic Pathobiological Aspects and Therapeutc Appro*, Vol.14, No.2, pp. 81-90, ISSN 1073-2322.

Bahrani-Mougeot, FK., Paster, BJ., Coleman, S., Ashar, J., Knost, S., Sautter, RL., & Lockhart, PB. (2008). Identification of oral bacteria in blood cultures by conventional *versus* molecular methods. *Oral Surgery, Oral Medicine, Oral Pathology, Oral Radiology, and Endodontics*, Vol.105, No.6, pp.720-724, ISSN 1079-2104.

Baltch, AL., Pressman, HL., Hammer, MC., Sutphen, NC., Smith, RP., & Shayegani, M. (1982). Bacteremia following dental extractions in patients with and without penicillin prophylaxis. *American Journal of the Medical Sciences*, Vol.283, No.3, pp.129-140, ISSN 0002-9629.

Barbosa, M., Carmona, IT., Amaral, B., Limeres, J., Álvarez, M., Cerqueira, C., & Diz, P. (2010). General anesthesia increases the risk of bacteremia following dental extractions. *Oral Surgery, Oral Medicine, Oral Pathology, Oral Radiology, and Endodontics*, Vol.110, No.6, pp.706-712, ISSN 1079-2104.

Beck, J., García, R., Heiss, G., Vokonas, PS., & Offenbacher S. (1996). Periodontal disease and cardiovascular disease. *Journal of Periodontology*, Vol.67, Suppl.10, pp.1123-1137, ISSN 0022-3492.

Bender, IB, & Pressman, RS. (1945). Factors in dental bacteremia. *Journal of the American Dental Association,* Vol.32, No.1, pp.836-853, ISSN 0002-8177.

Bender, IB., Seltzer, S., & Yermish, M. (1960). The incidence of bacteremia in endodontic manipulation: preliminary report. *Oral Surgery, Oral Medicine, and Oral Pathology,* Vol. 13, pp.353-360, ISSN 0030-4220.

Bender, IB., Seltzer, S., Tashman S., & Meloff, G. (1963). Dental procedures in patients with rheumatic heart disease. *Oral Surgery, Oral Medicine and Oral Pathology,* Vol.16, pp.466-473, ISSN 0030-4220.

Berger, SA., Weitzman, S., Edberg, SC., & Casey, JI. (1974). Bacteremia after the use of an oral irrigation device. A controlled study in subjects with normal-appearing gingiva: comparison with use of toothbrush. *Annals of Internal Medicine,* Vol.80, No.4, pp.510-511, ISSN 0003-4819.

Bernstein, M. (1932). Subacute bacterial endocarditis following the extraction of teeth: report of a case. *Annals of Internal Medicine,* Vol.5, No.9, pp.1138-1144, ISSN 0003-4819.

Bhanji, S., Williams, B., Sheller, B., Elwood, T., & Mancl, L. (2002). Transient bacteremia induced by toothbrushing: a comparison of the Sonicare toothbrush with a conventional toothbrush. *Pediatric Dentistry,* Vol.24, No.4, pp.295-299, ISSN 0164-1263.

Billings, F. (1909). Chronic infectious endocarditis. *Archives of Internal Medicine,* Vol.4, No.5, pp.409-431, ISSN 0003-9926.

Billings, F. (1912). Chronic focal infections and their etiologic relations to arthritis and nephritis. *Archives of Internal Medicine,* Vol.9, No.4, pp.484-498, ISSN 0003-9926.

Billings, F. (1916). *Focal infection: The Lane Medical Lectures,* D. Appleton and Company, New York.

Brennan, MT., Kent, ML., Fox, PC., Norton, HJ., & Lockhart, PB. (2007). The impact of oral disease and nonsurgical treatment on bacteremia in children. *Journal of the American Dental Association,* Vol.138, No.1, pp.80-85, ISSN 0002-8177.

Bristish Cardiac Society Clinical Practice Committee & Royal College of Physicians. (2004). Dental aspects of endocarditis prophylaxis: new recommendations from a Working Group of the Bristish Cardiac Society Clinical Practice Committee and Royal College of Physicians Clinical Effectiveness and Evaluation, In: *Bristish Cardiac Society Clinical Practice Committee & Royal College of Physicians,* July 2010, Available from: < http://www.bcs.com/library>.

Brown, HH. (1932). Tooth extraction and chronic infective endocarditis. *British Medical Journal,* Vol.1, No.3721, pp.796-797, ISSN 0007-1447.

Burden, DJ., Coulter, WA., Johnston, CD., Mullally, B., & Stevenson, M. (2004). The prevalence of bacteraemia on removal of fixed orthodontic appliances. *European Journal of Orthodontics,* Vol.26, No.4, pp.443-447, ISSN 0141-5387.

Burket, LW., & Burn CG. (1937). Bacteremias following dental extraction. Demonstration of source of bacteria by means of a non-pathogen (*Serratia marcescens*). *Journal of Dental Research,* Vol.16, pp.521-530, ISSN 0022-0345.

Carmona, IT., Diz-Dios, P., & Scully, C. (2002). An update on the controversies in bacterial endocarditis of oral origin. *Oral Surgery, Oral Medicine, Oral Pathology, Oral Radiology, and Endodontics,* Vol.93, No.6, pp.660-670, ISSN 1079-2104

Castillo, DM., Sánchez-Beltrán, MC., Castellanos, JE., Sanz, I., Mayorga-Fayad, I., Sanz, M., & Lafaurie, GI. (2011). Detection of specific periodontal microorganisms from bacteraemia samples after periodontal therapy using molecular-based diagnostics. *Journal of Clinical Periodontology,* Vol.38, No.5, pp.418-427, ISSN 0303-6979.

Chapin, K., & Lauderdale, TL. (1996). Comparison of Bactec 9240 and Difco ESP blood culture systems for detection of organisms from vials whose entry was delayed. *Journal of Clinical Microbiology,* Vol.34, No.3, pp.543-549, ISSN 0095-1137.

Cobe, HM. (1954). Transitory bacteremia. *Oral Surgery, Oral Medicine, and Oral Pathology,*Vol.7, No.6, pp.609-615, ISSN 0030-4220.

Cohen, DJ., Malave D., Ghidoni, JJ., Lakovidis, P., Everett, MM., You, S., Liu, Y., &, Boyan, BD. (2004). Role of oral bacterial flora in calcific aortic stenosis: an animal model. *The Annals of Thoracic Surgery,* Vol.77, No.2, pp. 537-543, ISSN 0003-4975.

Coulter, WA., Coffey, A., Saunders, ID., & Emmerson, AM. (1990). Bacteremia in children following dental extraction. *Journal of Dental Research,* Vol.69, No.10, pp.1691-1695, ISSN 0022-0345.

Crasta, K., Daly, CG., Mitchell, D., Curtis, B., Stewart, D., & Heitz-Mayfield, LJ. (2009). Bacteraemia due to dental flossing. *Journal of Clinical Periodontology,* Vol.36, No.4, pp.323-332, ISSN 0303-6979.

Dajani, AS., Taubert, KA., Wilson, W., Bolger, AF., Bayer, A., Ferrieri, P., Gewitz, MH., Shulman, ST., Nouri, S., Newburguer, JW., Hutto, C., Pallasch, TJ., Gage, TW., Levison, ME., Peter, G., & Zuccaro, G.Jr. (1997). Prevention of bacterial endocarditis. Recommendations by the American Heart Association. *Journal of the American Medical Association,* Vol.277, No.22, pp.1794-1801, ISSN 0098-7484.

Daly, C., Mitchell, D., Grossberg, D, Highfield, J., Stewart, D. (1997). Bacteraemia caused by periodontal probing. *Australian Dental Journal,* Vol.42, No.2, pp.77-80, ISSN 0045-0421.

De Leo, AA., Schoenknecht, FD., Anderson, MW., & Peterson, JC. (1974). The incidence of bacteremia following oral prophylaxis on pediatric patients. *Oral Surgery, Oral Medicine, and Oral Pathology* Vol.37, No.1; pp.36-45, ISSN 0030-4220.

Debelian, GJ., Olsen, I., & Tronstad, L. (1995). Bacteremia in conjunction with endodontic therapy. *Endodontics & Dental Traumatology,* Vol.11, No.3, pp.142-149, ISSN 0109-2502.

Degling, TE. (1972). Orthodontics, bacteremia, and the heart damaged patient. *The Angle Orthodontists,* Vol.42, No.4, pp. 399-402, ISSN 0003-3219.

Delahaye, F., & De Gevigney, G. (2001). Should we give antibiotic prophylaxis against infective endocarditis in all cardiac patients, whatever the type of dental treatment?. *Heart,* Vol.85, No.1, pp.9-10, ISSN 1355-6037.

DeStefano, F., Anda, RF., Kahn, HS., Williamson, DF., & Russell CM. (1993). Dental disease and risk of coronary heart disease. *British Medical Journal (Clinical Research ed.),* Vol.306, No.6879, pp.688-691, ISSN 0959-535X.

Dietrich, T., Jimenez, M., Krall-Kaye, EA., Vokonas, PS., & Garcia, RI. (2008). Age-dependent associations between chronic periodontitis/edentulism and risk of coronary heart disease. *Circulation,* Vol.117, No.13, pp.1668-1674, ISSN 0009-7322.

Diz, P., Tomás, I., & Limeres, J. (2011). Bacteremias producidas por intervenciones odontológicas, In: *Patología Periodontal y Cardiovascular. Su interrelación e implicaciones para la salud,* Sociedad Española de Periodoncia y Osteointegración and Sociedad Española de Cardiología, pp. 159-167, Editorial Médica Panamericana, ISBN 978-84-9835-313-6, Madrid.

Drangsholt, MT. A new causal model of dental diseases associated with endocarditis (1998). *Annals of Periodontology*; Vol.3, No.1, pp.184-196, ISSN 1553-0841.

Eachempati, SR., Hydo, L., & Barie, PS. (1999). Gender-based differences in outcome in patients with sepsis. *Archives of Surgery*, Vol.134, No.12, pp.1342-1347, ISSN 0004-0010.

Easlick, KA. (1951). An evaluation of the effect of dental foci of infection on health. *Journal of the American Dental Association*, Vol.42, No.6, pp.615-697, ISSN 0002-8177.

Elliott, RH., & Dunbar, JM. (1968). Streptococcal bacteraemia in children following dental extractions. *Archives of Disease in Childhood*, Vol.43, No.230, pp.451-454, ISSN 0003-9888.

Elliott, SD. (1939). Bacteraemia and oral sepsis. *Proceedings of the Royal Society of Medicine*,Vol.32, pp.747-754, ISSN 0035-9157.

Erverdi, N., Kadir, T., Özkan, H., & Acar, A. (1999). Investigation of bacteremia after orthodontic banding. *Amerian Journal of Orthodontics and Dentofacial Orthopedics*, Vol.116, No.6, pp.687-690, ISSN 0889-5406.

Feldman, L., & Trace, IM. (1938). Subacute bacterial endocarditis following the removal of teeth or tonsils. *Annals of Internal Medine*, Vol.11, No.12, pp.2124-2132, ISSN 0003-4819.

Felix, JE., Rosen, S., & App, GR. (1971). Detection of bacteremia after the use of an oral irrigation device in subjects with periodontitis. *Journal of Periodontology*, Vol.42, No.12, pp.785-787, ISSN 0022-3492.

Fine, DH., Furgang, D., McKiernan, M., Tereski-Bischio, D., Ricci-Nittel, D., Zhang, P., & Araujo, MW. (2010). An investigation of the effect of an essential oil mouthrinse on induced bacteraemia: a pilot study. *Journal of Clinical Periodontology*, Vol.37, No.9, pp.840-847, ISSN 0303-6979.

Fish, EW., & Maclean, I. (1936). The distribution of oral streptococci in the tissues. *British Dental Journal*,Vol.61, pp.336-362, ISSN 0007-0610.

Forner, L., Larsen, T., Kilian, M., & Holmstrup, P. (2006). Incidence of bacteremia after chewing, toothbrushing and scaling in individuals with periodontal inflammation. *Journal of Clinical Periodontology*, Vol.33, No.6, pp.401-407, ISSN 0303-6979.

Gaetti-Jardim, E Jr., Marcelino, SL., Feitosa, AC., Romito, GA., & Avila-Campos, MJ. (2009). Quantitative detection of periodontopathic bacteria in atherosclerotic plaques from coronary arteries. *Journal of Medical Microbiology*, Vol.58, No.12, pp.1568-1575, ISSN 0022-2615.

Geiger, AJ. (1942). Relation of fatal subacute bacterial endocarditis to tooth extraction. *Journal of the American Dental Association*, Vol.29, pp.1023-1025, ISSN 0002-8177.

Giglio, JA., Rowland, RW., Dalton, HP., & Laskin, DM. (1992). Suture removal-induced bacteremia: a possible endocarditis risk. *Journal of the American Dental Association*, Vol.123, No.8, pp.65-70, ISSN 0002-8177.

Gould, FK., Elliot, TS., Foweraker, J., Fulford, M., Perry, JD., Roberts, GJ., Sandoe, JA., Watkin, RW., & Working Party of the British Society for Antimicrobial Chemotherapy. (2006). Guidelines for the prevention of endocarditis: report of the Working Party of the British Society for Antimicrobial Chemotherapy. *Journal of Antimicrobial Chemotherapy*, Vol.57, No.6, pp.1035-1042, ISSN 0305-7453.

Guntheroth, WG. (1984). How important are dental procedures as a cause of infective endocarditis?. *The American Journal of Cardiology*, Vol.54, No.7, pp.797-801, ISSN 0002-9149.

Habib, G., Hoen, B., Tornos, P., Thuny, F., Prendergast, B., Vilacosta, I., Moreillon, P., de Jesus Antunes, M., Thilen, U., Lekakis, J., Lengyel, M., Müller, L., Naber, CK., Nihoyannopoulos, P., Moritz, A., Zamorano, JL., ESC Committee for Practice Guidelines., Vahanian, A., Auricchio, A., Bax, J., Ceconi, C., Dean, V., Filippatos, G., Funck-Brentano, C., Hobbs, R., Kearney, P., McDonagh, T., McGregor, K., Popescu, BA., Reiner, Z., Sechtem, U., Sirnes, PA., Tendera, M., Vardas, P., Widimsky, P, Vahanian. A., Aguilar, R., Bongiorni, MG., Borger, M., Butchart, E., Danchin, N., Delahaye, F., Erbel, R., Franzen, D., Gould, K., Hall, R., Hassager, C., Kjeldsen, K., McManus, R., Miró, JM., Mokracek, A., Rosenhek, R., San Román, JA., Seferonic, P., Selton-Suty, C., Sousa, M., Trinchero, R., & van Camp, G. (2009). Guidelines on the prevention, diagnosis, and treatment of infective endocarditis (new version 2009): the Task Force on the Prevention, Diagnosis, and Treatment of Infective Endocarditis of the European Society of Cardiology (ESC). Endorsed by the European Society of Clinical Microbiology and Infectious Disease (ESCMID) and the International Society of Chemotherapy (ISC) for Infection and Cancer. *European Heart Journal*, Vol.30, No.19. pp.2369-2413, ISSN 0195-668X.

Hall, G., Hedström, SA., Heimdahl, A., & Nord, CE. (1993). Prophylactic administration of penicillins for endocarditis does not reduce the incidence of postextraction bacteremia. *Clinical Infectious Disease*, Vol.17, No.2, pp.188-194, ISSN 1058-4838.

Hartzell, JD., Torres, D., Kim, P., & Wortmann, G. (2005). Incidence of bacteraemia after routine tooth brushing. *American Journal of the Medical Sciences*, Vol.329, No.4, pp.178-180, ISSN 0002-9629.

Heimdahl, A., Hall, G., Hedberg, M., Sandberg, H., Söder, PO., Tunér, K., & Nord, CE. (1990). Detection and quantitation by lysis-filtration of bacteremia after different oral surgical procedures. *Journal of Clinical Microbiology*, Vol.28, No.10, pp.2205-2209, ISSN 0095-1137.

Hirsh, HL., Vivino, JJ., Merril, A., & Dowling, HF. (1948). Effect of prophylactically administered penicillin on incidence of bacteremia following extraction of teeth; results in patients with healed rheumatic and bacterial endocarditis. *Archives of Internal Medicine*, Vol.81, No.6, pp.868-878, ISSN 0730-188X.

Holman, WL. (1928). Focal infection and "elective localization". *Archives of Pathology & Laboratory Medicine*, Vol.5, pp.68-136, ISSN 0003-9985.

Hopkins, JA. (1939). *Streptococcus viridans*: bacteremia following extraction of the teeth. *Journal of the American Dental Association*, Vol.26, pp.2002-2008, ISSN 0002-8177.

Hunter, W. (1900). Oral sepsis as a cause of disease. *British Medical Journal*, Vol.2, No.2065, pp. 215-216, ISSN 0007-1447.

Hupp, JR. (1993). Changing methods of preventing infective endocarditis following dental procedures: 1943-1993. *Journal of Oral and Maxillofacial Surgery*, Vol.51, No.6, pp. 616-623, ISSN 0278-2391.

Jones, DJ., Munro, CL., Grap, MJ., Kitten, T., & Edmond, M. (2010). Oral care and bacteremia risk in mechanically ventilated adults. *Heart & Lung: The Journal of Critical Care*, Vol.39, Suppl.6, pp.S57-S65, ISSN 0147-9563.

Jordan, JA., Jones-Laughner, J., & Durso, MB. (2009). Utility of pyrosequencing in identifying bacteria directly from positive blood culture bottles. *Journal of Clinical Microbiology*, Vol.47, No.2, pp.368-372, ISSN 0095-1137.

Josefsson, K., Heimdahl, A., von Konow, L., & Nord, CE. (1985). Effect of phenoxymethylpenicillin and erythromycin prophylaxis on anaerobic bacteraemia after oral surgery. *Journal of Antimicrobial Chemotherapy*, Vol.16, No.2, pp.243-251, ISSN 0305-7453.

Kelson, SR., & White, PD. (1945). Notes on 250 cases of subacute bacterial (streptococcal) endocarditis studied and treated between 1927 and 1939. *Annals of Internal Medicine,*Vol.22, No.1, pp.40-60, ISSN 0003-4819.

Keosian, J., Rafel, S., & Weinman, I. (1956). The effect of aqueous diatomic iodine mouthwashes on the incidence of postextraction bacteremia. *Oral Surgery, Oral Medicine, and Oral Pathology*, Vol.9, No.12, pp.1337-1341, ISSN 0030-4220.

Kinane, DF., Riggio, MP., Walker, KF., MacKenzie, D., & Shearer, B. (2005). Bacteremia following periodontal procedures. *Journal of Clinical Periodontology*, Vol.32, No.7, pp.708-713, ISSN 0303-6979.

Lafaurie, GI., Mayorga-Fayad, I., Torres, MF., Castillo, DM., Aya, MR., Barón, A., & Hurtado, PA. (2007). Periodontopathic microorganisms in peripheric blood after scaling and root planing. *Journal of Clinical Periodontology*, Vol.34, No.10, pp.873-879, ISSN 0303-6979.

Lineberger, LT., & De Marco, TJ. (1973). Evaluation of transient bacteremia following routine periodontal procedures. *Journal of Periodontology*, Vol.44, No.12, pp.757-762, ISSN 0022-3492.

Lockhart, PB., Brennan, MT., Thornhill, M., Michalowicz, BS., Noll, J., Bahrani-Mougeot, FK., & Sasser, HC. (2009) Poor oral hygiene as a risk factor for infective endocarditis-related bacteremia. *Journal of the American Dental Association*, Vol.140, No.10, pp.1238-1244, ISSN 0002-8177.

Lockhart, PB. (1996). An analysis of bacteremias during dental extractions. A doble-blind, placebo-controlled study of chlorhexidine. *Archives of Internal Medicine*, Vol.156, No.5, pp.513-520, ISSN 0003-9926.

Lockhart, PB., Brennan, MT., Sasser, HC., Fox, PC., Paster, BJ., & Bahrani-Mougeot, FK. (2008). Bacteremia associated with toothbrushing and dental extraction. *Circulation*, Vol.117, No.24, pp.3118-3125, ISSN 0009-7322.

Lofthus, JE., Waki, MY., Jolkovsky, DL., Otomo-Corgel, J., Newman, MG., Flemming, T., & Nachnani, S. (1991). Bacteremia following subgingival irrigation and scaling and root planing. *Journal of Periodontology*, Vol.62, No.10, pp. 602-607, ISSN 0022-3492.

Loza Fernández de Bobadilla, E., Planes, A., & Rodríguez, M. (2003). Procedimientos en Microbiología Clínica. Recomendaciones de la Sociedad Española de Enfermedades Infecciosas y Microbiología Clínica. 3a Hemocultivos, In: *Sociedad Española de Enfermedades Infecciosas en Microbiología Clínica*, July 2010, Available from: <http://www.seimc.org/documentos/protocolos/microbiologia/>

Lucas, VS., & Roberts, GJ. (2000). Odontogenic bacteremia following tooth cleaning procedures in children. *Pediatric Dentistry*, Vol.22, No.2, pp.96-100, ISSN 0164-1263.

Lucas, VS., Gafan, G., Dewhurst, S., & Roberts, GJ. (2008). Prevalence, intensity and nature of bacteremia after toothbrushing. *Journal of Dentistry*, Vol.36, No.7, pp.481-487, ISSN 0300-5712.

Lucas, VS., Kyriazidou, A., Gelbier, M., & Roberts, GJ. (2007). Bacteraemia following debanding and gold chain adjustment. *European Journal of Orthodontics*, Vol.29, No.2, pp. 161-165, ISSN 0141-5387.

Lucas, VS., Lytra, V., Hassan, T., Tatham, H., Wilson, M., & Roberts, GJ. (2002a). Comparison of lysis filtration and an automated blood culture system (BACTEC) for detection, quantification, and identification of odontogenic bacteremia in children. *Journal of Clinical Microbiology,* Vol.40, No.9, pp.3416-3420, ISSN 0095-1137.

Lucas, VS., Omar, J., Vieira, A., & Roberts, GJ. (2002b). The relationship between odontogenic bacteraemia and orthodontic treatment procedures. *European Journal of Orthodontics,* Vol.24, No.3, pp.293-301, ISSN 0141-5387.

Madsen, KL. (1974). Effect of chlorhexidine mouthrinse and periodontal treatment upon bacteremia produced by oral hygiene procedures. *Scandinavian Journal of Dental Research,* Vol.82, No.1, pp.1-7, ISSN 0022-0345.

Maestre, JR., Mateo, M., & Sánchez, P. (2008). Bacteremia secundaria a procedimientos odontológicos periodontales. *Revista Española de Quimioterapia,* Vo.21. No.3, pp.153-156, ISSN 0214-3429.

McLaughlin, JO., Coulter, WA., Coffey, A., & Burden DJ. (1996). The incidence of bacteremia after orthodontic banding. *American Journal of Orthodontics and Dentofacial Orthopedics,* Vol.109, pp.639-644, ISSN 0889-5406.

Misra, S., Percival, RS., Devine, DA., & Duggal, MS. (2007). A pilot study to assess bacteremia associated with tooth brushing using conventional, electric or ultrasonic toothbrushes. *European Archives of Paediatric Dentistry,* Vol.8, Suppl.1, pp.42-45, ISSN 1818-6300.

Monteiro, AM., Jardini, MA., Alves, S., Giampaoli, V., Aubin, EC., Figueiredo-Neto, AM., & Gidlund, M. (2009). Cardiovascular disease parameters in periodontitis. *Journal of Periodontology,* Vol.80, No.3, pp.378-388, ISSN 0022-3492.

Murphy, AM., Daly, CG., Mitchell, DH., Stewart, D., & Curtis, BH. (2006). Chewing fails to induce oral bacteraemia in patients with periodontal disease. *Journal of Clinical Periodontology,* Vol.33, No.10, pp.730-736, ISSN 0303-6979.

Murray, M., & Moosnick, BS. (1941). Incidence of bacteremia in patients with dental disease. *Journal of Laboratory and Clinical Medicine,* Vol.26, pp.801-802, ISSN 0022-2143.

Nakano, K., Nemoto, H., Nomura, R., Inaba, H., Yoshioka, H., Taniguchi, K., Amano, A., & Ooshima, T. (2009). Detection of oral bacteria in cardiovascular specimens. *Oral Microbiology and Immunology,* Vol.24, No.1, pp.64-68, ISSN 0902-0055.

National Institute for Health and Clinical Excellence. (2008). Prophylaxis against infective endocarditis, In: *National Institute for Health and Clinical Excellence,* July 2010, Available from: http://www.nice.org.uk/nicemedia/pdf/PIEGuidelines.pdf.

Northrop, PM., & Crowley, MC. (1943). The prophylactic use of sulfathiazole in transient bacteremia following extraction of teeth. *Journal of Oral Surgery,* Vol.1, pp.19-29, ISSN 0022-3255.

Offner, PJ., Moore, EE., & Biffl, WL. (1999). Male gender is a risk factor for major infections after surgery. *Archives of Surgery,* Vol.134, No.9, pp.935-940, ISSN 0004-0010.

Okabe, K., Nakagawa, K., & Yamamoto, E. (1995). Factors affecting the occurrence of bacteremia associated with tooth extraction. *International Journal of Oral and Maxillofacial Surgery,* Vol.24, No.3, pp.239-242, ISSN 0901-5027.

Okell, CC., & Elliott, SD. (1935). Bacteremia and oral sepsis with special reference to the aetiology of subacute endocarditis. *Lancet;* Vol.2, pp.869-872, ISSN 0140-6736.

Olsen, I. (2008). Update on bacteraemia related to dental procedures. *Transfusion and Apheresis Science,* Vol.39, No.2, pp. 173-178, ISSN 1473-0502.

Onçag, O., Aydemir, S., Ersin, N., & Koca, H. (2006). Bacteremia incidence in pediatric patients under dental general anesthesia. *Congenital Heart Disease,* Vol.1, No.5, pp.224-228, ISSN 1747-079X.

Pallasch, TJ. (2003). Antibiotic prophylaxis: problems in paradise. *Dental Clinics of North America*, Vol.47, No.4, pp.665-79, ISSN 0011-8532

Palmer, HD., & Kempf, M. (1939). *Streptococcus viridans* bacteremia following extraction of teeth: a case of multiple mycotic aneurysms in the pulmonary arteries: report of cases and necropsies. *Journal of the American Medical Association*, Vol.113, No.20, pp.1788-1792, ISSN 0098-7484.

Parahitiyawa, NB., Jin, LJ., Leung, WK., Yam, WC., & Samaranayake, P. (2009). Microbiology of odontogenic bacteremia: beyond endocarditis. *Clinical Microbiology Reviews*, Vol.22, No.1, pp. 46-64, ISSN 0893-8512.

Pérez-Chaparro, PJ., Gracieux, P., Lafaurie, GI., Donnio, PY., & Bonnaure-Mallet, M. (2008). Genotypic characterization of *Porphyromonas gingivalis* isolated from subgingival plaque and blood sample in positive bacteremia subjects with periodontitis. *Journal of Clinical Periodontology*, Vol.35, No.9, pp.748-753, ISSN 0303-6979.

Peterson, LJ., & Peacock, R. (1976). The incidence of bacteremia in pediatric patients following tooth extraction. *Circulation*, Vol. 53, No.4, pp.676-679, ISSN 0009-7322.

Piñeiro, A., Tomás, I., Blanco, J., Álvarez, M., Seoane, J., & Diz, P. (2010). Bacteraemia following dental implants' placement. *Clinical Oral Implants Research*, Vol.21, No.9, pp.913-918, ISSN 0905-7161.

Pucar, A., Milasin, J., Lekovic, V., Vukadinovic, M., Ristic, M., Putnik, S., & Kenney, EB. (2007). Correlation between atherosclerosis and periodontal putative pathogenic bacterial infections in coronary and internal mammary arteries. *Journal of Periodontology*, Vol.78, No.4, pp.677-682, ISSN 0022-3492.

Ramadan, AE., Zaki, SA., & Nour, ZM. (1975). A study of transient bacteraemia following the use of dental floss silk and interdental stimulators. *Egyptian Dental Journal*, Vol. 21, No.4, pp.19-28, ISSN 0070-9484.

Reimann, HA., & Havens, WP. (1940). Focal infection and systemic disease: a critical appraisal. The case against indiscriminate removal of teeth and tonsils clinical lecture at St. Louis Session. *Journal of the American Medical Association*, Vol.114, No.1, pp.1-6, ISSN 0098-7484.

Reinhardt, RA., Bolton, RW., & Hlava, G. (1982). Effect of nonsterile *versus* sterile water irrigation with ultrasonic scaling on postoperative bacteremias. *Journal of Periodontology*, Vol.53, No.2, pp.96-100, ISSN 0022-3492.

Rhoads, PS., Schram, WR., & Adair, D. (1950). Bacteremia following tooth extraction: prevention with penicillin and N U 445. *Journal of the American Dental Association*, Vol.41, No.1, pp.55-61, ISSN 0002-8177.

Richards, JH. (1932). Bacteremia following irritation of foci of infection. *Journal of the American Medical Association*, Vol.99, No.18, pp.1496-1497, ISSN 0098-7484.

Roberts, G., Gardner, P., & Simmons, N. (1992). Optimum sampling time for detection of dental bacteraemia in children. *International Journal of Cardiology* Vol.35, No.3; pp.311-315. ISSN 0167-5273

Roberts, GJ. (1999). Dentists are innocent! "Everyday" bacteremia is the real culprit: a review and assessment of the evidence that dental surgical procedures are a principal cause of bacterial endocarditis in children. *Pediatric Cardiology*, Vol.20, No.5, pp.317-325, ISSN 0172-0643.

Roberts, GJ., Gardner, P., Longhurst, P., Black, AE., & Lucas, VS. (2000). Is there a need for antibiotic prophylaxis for some aspects of paediatric conservative dentistry?. *British Dental Journal*, Vol.188, No.2, pp.95-98, ISSN 0007-0610.

Roberts, GJ., Holzel, HS., Sury, MR., Simmons, NA., Gardner, P., & Longhurst, P. (1997). Dental bacteremia in children. *Pediatric Cardiology*, Vol.18, No.1, pp.24-27, ISSN 0172-0643.

Roberts, GJ., Jaffray, EC., Spratt, DA., Petrie, A., Greville, C., Wilson, M., & Lucas, VS. (2006). Duration, prevalence and intensity of bacteraemia after dental extractions in children. *Heart*, Vol.92, No.9, pp.1274-1277, ISSN 1355-6037.

Roberts, GJ., Simmons, NB., Longhurst, P., & Hewitt, PB. (1998a). Bacteraemia following local anaesthetic injections in children. *British Dental Journal*, Vol.185, No.6, pp.295-298, ISSN 0007-0610.

Roberts, GJ., Watts, R., Longhurst, P., & Gardner P. (1998b). Bacteremia of dental origin and antimicrobial sensitivity following oral surgical procedures in children. *Pediatric Dentistry*, Vol.20, No.1, pp.28-36, ISSN 0164-1263.

Robinson, L., Kraus, FW., Lazansky, JP., Wheeler, RE., Gordon, S., & Johnson, V. (1950). Bacteremias of dental origin. II. A study of the factors influencing occurrence and detection. *Oral Surgery, Oral Medicine, and Oral Pathology*, Vol.3, pp.923-926, ISSN 0030-4220.

Romans, AR, & App, GR. (1971). Bacteremia, a result from oral irrigation in subjects with gingivitis. *Journal of Periodontology*, Vol.42, No.12, pp.757-760, ISSN 0022-3492.

Romero, J., Bouza, E., Loza, E., Planes, A., Rodríguez, A. (1993). *Procedimientos en Microbiología Clínica. Recomendaciones de la Sociedad Española de Enfermedades Infecciosas y Microbiología Clínica. 3 Hemocultivos*, In: Sociedad Española de Enfermedades Infecciosas en Microbiología Clínica, July 2010, Available from: <http://www.seimc.org/documentos/protocolos/microbiologia/>

Rosenow, EC. (1914). Transmutations within the *Streptococcus-Pneumococcus* group. *Journal of Infectious Disease*, Vol.14, No.1, pp.1-32, ISSN 0022-1899.

Savarrio, L., Mackenzie, D., Riggio, M., Saunders, WP., & Bagg, J. (2005). Detection of bacteraemias during non-surgical root canal treatment. *Journal of Dentistry*, Vol.33, No.4, pp.293-303, ISSN 0300-5712.

Schlegel, D., Reichart, PA., & Pfaff, U. (1978). Experimental bacteremia to demonstrate the barrier function of epithelium and connective tissue surrounding oral endosseous implants. *International Journal of Oral Surgery*, Vol.7, No.6, pp.569-572, ISSN 0300-9785.

Schlein, RA., Kudlick, EM., Reindorf, CA., Gregory, J., & Royal, GC. (1991). Toothbrushing and transient bacteraemia in patients undergoing orthodontic treatment. *American Journal of Orthodontics and Dentofacial Orthopedics*, Vol.99, No.5, pp.466-472, ISSN 0889-5406.

Sconyers, JR., Crawford, JJ., & Moriarty, JD. (1973). Relationship of bacteremia to toothbrushing in patients with periodontitis. *Journal of the American Dental Association*, Vol.87, No.3, pp.616-622, ISSN 0002-8177.

Seymour, RA., Lowry, R., Whitworth, JM., & Martin, MV. (2000). Infective endocarditis, dentistry and antibiotic prophylaxis; time for a rethink?. *British Dental Journal*, Vol.189, No.11, pp.610-616, ISSN 0007-0610.

Shanson, DC., Cannon, P., & Wilks, M. (1978). Amoxycillin compared with penicillin V for the prophylaxis of dental bacteraemia. *The Journal of the Antimicrobial Chemotherapy*, Vol.4, No.5, pp.431-436, ISSN 0305-7453.

Silver, JG., Martin, AW., & McBride, BC. (1977). Experimental transient bacteraemias in human subjects with varying degrees of plaque accumulation and gingival inflammation. *Journal of Clinical Periodontology*, Vol.4, No.2. pp.92-99, ISSN 0303-6979.

Sonbol, H., Spratt, D., Roberts, GJ., & Lucas, VS. (2009). Prevalence, intensity, and identity of bacteraemia following conservative dental procedures in children. *Oral Microbiology and Immnunology*, Vol.24, No.3, pp.177-182, ISSN 0902-0055.

Speck, WT., Spear, SS., Krongrad, E., Mandel, L., & Gersony, WM. (1976). Transient bacteremia in pediatric patients after dental extraction. *American Journal of Diseases of Children*, Vol.130, No.4, pp.406-407, ISSN 0002-922X.

Stein, JM., Kuch, B., Conrads, G., Fickl, S., Chrobot, J., Schulz, S., Ocklenburg, C., & Smeets, R. (2009). Clinical periodontal and microbiologic parameters in patients with acute myocardial infarction. *Journal of Periodontology*, Vol.80, No.10, pp.1581-1589, ISSN 0022-3492.

Takai, S., Kuriyama, T., Yanagisawa, M., Nakagawa, K., & Karasawa, T. (2005). Incidence and bacteriology of bacteremia associated with various oral and maxillofacial surgical procedures. *Oral Surgery, Oral Medicine, Oral Pathology, Oral Radiology, and Endodontics*, Vol.99, No.3, pp.292-298, ISSN 1079-2104.

Tamimi, HA., Thomassen, PR., & Moser, EH Jr. (1969). Bacteremia study using a water irrigation device. *Journal of Periodontology*, Vol.40, No.7, pp.4-6, ISSN 0022-3492.

Thomas, CB., France, R., & Reichsman F. (1941). Prophylactic use of sulfanilamide. In patients susceptible to rheumatic fever. *Journal of the American Medical Association*, Vol.116, No.7, pp.551-560, ISSN 0098-7484.

Tomás, I., Álvarez, M., Limeres, J., Potel, C., Medina, J., & Diz, P. (2007). Prevalence, duration and aetiology of bacteraemia following dental extractions. *Oral Diseases*, Vol.13, No.1, pp.56-62, ISSN 1354-523X.

Tomás, I., Diz, P., Tobías, A., Scully, C., & Donos N. (2011). Periodontal health status and bacteremia from daily oral activities: systematic review/meta-analysis. *Journal of Clinical Periodontology*, (in press), ISSN 0303-6979.

Wilson, W., Taubert, KA., Gewitz, M., Lockhart, PB., Baddour, LM., Levison, M., Bolger, A., Cabell, CH., Takahashi, M., Baltimore, RS., Newburger, JW., Strom, BL., Tani, LY., Gerber, M., Bonow, RO., Pallasch, T., Shulman, ST., Rowley, AH., Burns, JC., Ferrieri, P., Gardner, T., Goff, D., Durack, DT., American Heart Association Rheumatic Fever, Endocarditis and Kawasaki Disease Committee., American Heart Association and Council on Cardiovascular Disease in the Young., American Heart Association Council on Clinical Cardiology., American Heart Association Council on Cardiovascular Surgery and Anesthesia., & Quality of Care and Outcomes Research Interdisciplinary Working Group. (2007). Prevention of infective endocarditis: guidelines from the American Heart Association: a guideline from the American Heart Association Rheumatic Fever, Endocarditis, and Kawasaki Disease Committee, Council on Cardiovascular Disease in the Young, and the Council on Clinical Cardiology, Council on Cardiovascular Surgery and Anesthesia, and the Quality of Care and Outcomes Research Interdisciplinary Working Group. *Circulation*, Vol.116, No.15, pp.1736-1754, ISSN 0009-7322.

Witzenberger, T., O'Leary, TJ., & Gillette, WB. (1982). Effect of a local germicide on the occurrence of bacteremia during subgingival scaling. *Journal of Periodontology*, Vol.53, No.3, pp.172-179, ISSN 0022-3492.

Yanke, SJ., Olson, ME., Davies, HD., & Hart, DA. (2000). A CD-1 mouse model of infection with *Staphylococcus aureus*: influence of gender on infection with MRSA and MSSA isolates. *Canadian Journal of Microbiology*, Vol.46, No.10, pp.920-926, ISSN 0008-4166.

3

Platelet-Bacterial Interactions as Therapeutic Targets in Infective Endocarditis

Steven W. Kerrigan and Dermot Cox
Royal College of Surgeons in Ireland
Dublin,
Ireland

1. Introduction

Endocarditis is an inflammation of the lining of the heart and valves. It can be due to a non-infectious cause (Asopa et al., 2007) but when the inflammation is associated with an infection, usually bacterial, it is known as infective endocarditis (IE) and is characterized by the development of a large septic thrombus on one of the cardiac valves (Beynon et al., 2006; Moreillon and Que, 2004). As this thrombus grows, it can lead to valve failure or may fragment forming a septic embolus that is associated with high mortality if the target of the embolus is the brain, heart or lung (Homma and Grahame-Clarke, 2003). Untreated the mortality is very high and even with aggressive therapy with antibiotics and valve replacement surgery there is a significant mortality. Primarily the disease is due to the formation of a platelet-bacteria thrombus on a cardiac valve and this review will look at the interaction between bacteria and platelets within the context of endocarditis.

2. Traditional role of platelets in thrombosis

Platelets are anucleate fragments of megakaryocytes and their primary role is in haemostasis. Damage to the endothelium surrounding blood vessels leads to the exposure of the sub-endothelial layer that is rich in collagen and immobilised plasma proteins such as von Willebrand factor (vWf). Platelets bind to the newly exposed collagen and become activated. Many blood vessels, such as the coronary arteries are high shear vessels and the blood is flowing too fast to allow the platelets to bind to the collagen. However, under these high shear conditions immobilised vWf can interact with platelet GPIb, which slows down the platelets allowing them to subsequently interact with collagen. Once activated platelets aggregate to form a thrombus which the damaged blood vessel. GPIIb/IIIa mediates platelet aggregation by binding plasma fibrinogen, which as a divalent protein can bind to two separate GPIIb/IIIa molecules. As a result, activated platelets are cross-linked by fibrinogen, which forms the aggregates that seal the damaged vessel.

Platelets are highly responsive and can be activated by many different agonists. As well as two different collagen receptors ($\alpha2\beta1$ and GPVI) and two ADP receptors P_2X_1 and P_2Y_{12}, a serotonin receptor, an adrenergic receptor and a thromboxane A_2 receptor there are also three thrombin receptors (Protease-activated receptor (PAR)-1, GPIbα and PAR-4). Platelet activation is dependent on the sum of the signals from all of these receptors and not on any specific receptor. Signalling from these receptors is either phospholipase A_2/cyclooxygenase (COX)-mediated, resulting in the generation of thromboxane A_2, or protein kinase C-mediated. In contrast, the generation of intracellular cAmp in response to prostacylin binding to its receptor acts to inhibit platelet activation.

Aside from their ability to adhere to sites of damage and to form aggregates, platelets also secrete their granule contents in response to activation. Platelets contain three different granules: α-granules, dense granules and lysosomes. Dense granules are rich in small molecules especially ATP/ADP and serotonin, α-granules contain numerous plasma proteins typically associated with haemostasis and the lysosomes contain acid hydrolases. These secreted products act to enhance haemostasis as ADP activates other platelets, serotonin causes vasoconstriction and the secreted proteins support platelet aggregation.

3. The role of platelets in innate immunity

The biological role of platelets is not confined to haemostasis as platelets also play an important role in the innate immune system (Cox et al., 2011; Semple and Freedman, 2010). Platelets are ideally suited to this as they are present at very high concentration in the blood and are the first responders to any damage to the vasculature, which is the primary mechanism by which pathogens gain entry to the blood. To facilitate this, platelets contain surface receptors that allow it to respond to pathogens. Platelets contain pattern recognition receptors, especially Toll-like receptors (TLRs). These and other receptors (see below) allow platelets to respond to pathogens. As with other platelet agonists, platelets respond to pathogens by adhering to them and subsequently become activated leading to thrombus formation and secretion. In the context of the innate immune system, secretion is the primary response. Activated platelets secrete anti-microbial peptides that act to kill bacteria (Mercier et al., 2004). They also secrete cytokines such as CD40L and RANTES (Antczak et al., 2010) that act to recruit and activate a variety of immune cells to deal with the invading microorganism. Thus, platelets play a key role in the innate immune system where they directly act to kill bacteria as well as coordinating the response of the immune system to the pathogens.

4. The role of platelets in infective endocarditis

IE arises when the bacteria subvert the platelet response to infection and as a result, platelets become part of the pathogenic process. In IE the platelets interact with the bacteria and become activated. They secrete anti-microbial peptides but the bacteria are resistant. Once activated the platelets aggregate resulting in the formation of a platelet-bacteria aggregate. Not only are the bacteria resistant to the anti-bacterial peptides (Bayer et al., 1998; Fowler et al., 2000), they become surrounded by platelets and are able to evade immune surveillance. To further complicate matters even if the bacteria are susceptible to antibiotics, many antibiotics have poor penetration into the thrombus despite adequate plasma levels making treatment more difficult.

While the list of pathogens that have been known to cause IE is long (Baddour et al., 2005), the vast majority of cases with an identified pathogen are due to Staphylococci (primarily *S. aureus*) or Streptococci (primarily *S. sanguinis and S. oralis*). However, around 25% of IE cases are culture negative with no bacteria isolated from the blood (Naber and Erbel, 2007). There are a number of reasons for the failure to culture any organisms such as commencement of antibiotic therapy prior to obtaining the blood sample, infection with a fastidious bacterium or a non-bacterial (e.g., fungal) endocarditis. In this review we will focus on the mechanism of platelet activation by Staphylococci and Streptococci as not only are they the dominant species involved in IE but they are also the best studied. While even different strains of a bacterial species differ in their ability to interact with platelets some general principles can be seen which is important in devising new treatment strategies.

5. Platelet-bacterial interactions: General observations

There are three different types of interaction between platelets and bacteria. The first is an inherent ability of platelet receptors to recognise bacterial surface components. Alternatively, plasma proteins can bind to bacteria and these proteins can in turn bind to a platelet receptor. Typically these are acute phase reactants such as fibrinogen and complement. A third mechanism for interacting with platelets is the secretion of bacterial products or toxins that interact with platelets. The binding of platelets to bacteria either through a direct interaction or via a bridging protein can mediate platelet adhesion and/or platelet activation. Interactions with bacterial toxins leads to either platelet lysis or platelet activation. Typically bacterial proteins that mediate adhesion are distinct from those that mediate aggregation. Thus, bacteria can support platelet adhesion and/or trigger platelet activation. During sepsis the primary interaction between platelets and bacteria is platelet activation and is mediated by both toxin secretion and a direct interaction with the bacteria. However, infective endocarditis is a focal infection of a damaged heart valve. The initial step is mediated by adhesion to the damaged valve as well as subsequent adhesion of platelets to the immobilised bacteria. This adhesive interaction is important in ensuring that the bacteria and thrombus remain attached to the valve despite the presence of turbulent flow conditions. For IE to develop the initial adhesive interaction must be followed by activation of the platelets leading to platelet recruitment and growth of the thrombus. Most bacteria can interact with platelets through multiple mechanisms making it difficult to identify the roles of the different proteins (both bacterial and platelet) and is further complicated by interactions that are not only species-specific but strain-specific as well.

6. Platelet-bacterial interactions: The Staphylococcus

Regardless of the modern advances in antimicrobial therapy and surgical intervention *Staphylococcus aureus* is still the most frequent etiologic microorganism found in Infective endocarditis (Rasmussen et al., 2011). Its interaction with platelets is well characterised. Much of the investigations to date have focused on two separate but related features of this relationship; 1) toxins and 2) cell wall protein mediators of platelet activation (Table 1).

S. aureus is known to secrete several extracellular toxins. Alpha (α)-toxin is a 34 kDa toxin composed of 293 amino acids (Bernheimer, 1965). It is produced by almost all strains of *S. aureus*. Its expression is accessory-gene regulon (agr)-regulated and is secreted into the extracellular environment as a monomeric water soluble protein (Ikigai and Nakae, 1985). The toxin disrupts the cell membranes by binding to the lipid bilayer, forming an oligomeric structure that forms a water filled transmembrane pore (Valeva et al., 1996). Studies have demonstrated that the toxin has primarily two modes of interaction with host cells. These include binding specifically to the host target at low concentrations and non-specific adsorption to host target cell membranes at higher concentrations (Hildebrand et al., 1991).

Siegel and Cohen were the first to demonstrate that addition of α-toxin to human platelet-rich plasma induced platelets to undergo shape change and aggregation (Siegel and Cohen, 1964). In this study the authors demonstrated that platelets leaked their intracellular ions NAD⁺, K⁺ and ATP but not protein, into the surrounding environment thus concluding that the platelets were not being lysed. Additional studies demonstrated that when platelets were treated with α-toxin it caused them to swell but there were no clear signs of platelet lysis by electron microscopy (Bernheimer and Schwartz, 1965; Manohar et al., 1967). Further investigations into the molecular mechanism through which platelets became activated, found that pore formation gave rise to an increase in intracellular calcium concentration (Arvand et al., 1990; Baliakina et al., 1999). Arvand et al demonstrated that α-toxin triggers a platelet signal that leads to secretion of intracellular contents including procoagulant mediators, platelet factor 4 and factor V. Secreted factor V in turn associates with the platelet membrane leading to assembly of the prothrombinase complex (Arvand et al., 1990). This explains the major pathway responsible for the procoagulatory effects of α-toxin. Bayer et al. used 2 models to investigate the role of α-toxin on platelets. In the first and consistent with the above observations, the authors demonstrated that α-toxin caused platelet lysis which in turn caused the release of platelet microbial proteins (PMP's). The release of PMPs from platelets was bactericidal to *S. aureus*. Using an animal model of endocarditis the authors demonstrated that different strains of *S. aureus* differed in the expression of functional versus mutant forms of α-toxin. Under these conditions, the *S. aureus* strains producing either minimal or no α-toxin were less virulent in vivo than wild-type strains (Bayer et al., 1997). Wild-type *S. aureus* strains or indeed an isogenic strain engineered to over-express α-toxin were associated with increased release of PMP from platelets. These results suggest that when *S. aureus* releases α-toxin in the vicinity of platelets it triggers them to release of PMP's and therefore forging a protective role for the host by destroying the α-toxin producing *S. aureus*.

Lipoteichoic acid (LTA) is a component of gram positive bacteria (Morath et al., 2005) and is often released from the bacteria upon lysis or after treatment with β-lactam antibiotics (Lotz et al., 2006). It also stimulates a strong immune response through an interaction with toll like receptors expressed on many host cells (Zahringer et al., 2008). Toll like receptor 2 (TLR2) recognises LTA and there are now many reports in the literature demonstrating that TLR2 is expressed and functional on platelets (Blair et al., 2009; Keane et al., 2010b; Kerrigan et al., 2008; Ward et al., 2005) suggesting that platelets can respond to LTA. Early reports demonstrated that *S. aureus* LTA inhibits platelet activation by activating the cyclic AMP pathway (Sheu et al., 2000a; Sheu et al., 2000b).

S. aureus predominantly uses multiple cell wall surface proteins to interact with platelets to trigger their activation. Early studies by Hawiger et al. demonstrated that *S. aureus* cell wall protein A acts as a receptor for specific anti-staphylococcal antibodies which in turn bind FcγRIIa on platelets (Hawiger et al., 1979). This interaction triggers an intracellular signal that leads to granule release and platelet aggregation. While this interaction is important, deletion of protein A failed to abolish *S. aureus* binding to platelets. This observation suggests that other interactions between *S. aureus* and platelets exist.

Clumping factor A (ClfA) is a 97kDa protein has been shown to bind plasma fibrinogen. A mutant of *S. aureus* lacking clumping factor A (ClfA) failed to adhere to platelets, suggesting that ClfA binds fibrinogen which in turn binds the platelet fibrinogen receptor, GPIIbIIIa (Sullam et al., 1996). Further characterisation of this interaction suggested that ClfA also requires IgG in order to trigger platelet aggregation. Addition of fibrinogen and ClfA-specific immunoglobulin to the plasma-free system led to *S. aureus*-induced platelet aggregation. Even though resting GPIIbIIIa has little or no affinity for soluble fibrinogen it can still bind fibrinogen bound to bacteria, however this is not enough to trigger activation. To trigger full platelet activation both fibrinogen and specific immunoglobulin must bind to the A domain on ClfA. There are two distinct sites on ClfA that allows fibrinogen and IgG binding at the same time (Loughman et al., 2005). Once bound fibrinogen molecules can engage resting GPIIbIIIa, aided by bound ClfA specific immunoglobulin, which encourages the clustering of Fc receptor, FcγRIIa. This triggers activation of signal transduction leading to conformational change in GPIIbIIIa and aggregation of platelets.

Deletion of the fibrinogen binding domain (ClfA-PY) but not the IgG binding domain on ClfA led to the discovery of a second pathway S. *aureus* uses to induce platelet aggregation. By removing the fibrinogen binding domain in ClfA S. *aureus* induced platelet aggregation very slowly (between 8-20 minutes compared to 2-4 mins). These results suggest that IgG binding to ClfA alone is not enough to trigger platelet aggregation. Using a series of elimination experiments Loughman et al. demonstrated that complement must assemble on the S. *aureus* surface and then bind to unidentified complement receptors on the platelet. Therefore, in the absence of fibrinogen binding complement and specific immunoglobulin are required for platelet activation to occur (Loughman et al., 2005).

A major limitation in our current understanding of platelet bacterial interactions stems from the fact that the majority of studies cited in the literature to date have been carried out under static conditions (static adhesion assays) or non-physiological stirring conditions (platelet aggregation). Therefore, data obtained using *in vitro* assays may not be relevant to the fluid shear environment that platelets encounter in the vasculature. Indeed many reports suggests that the local fluid environment of the circulation critically affects the molecular pathways of cell-cell interactions (Varki, 1994). All of the early S. *aureus* studies were carried out under static or non-physiological stirring conditions and therefore it is difficult to relate these studies to the disease processes. Studies using a cone and plate viscometer (a device that shears cells at a given flow rate) have demonstrated that protein A, ClfA, SdrC, SdrD and SdrE are important in thrombus formation (George et al., 2007; George et al., 2006; Pawar et al., 2004). However, extremely high shear rates were used in these rheological studies. Using another method of investigating the influence of shear rates on S. *aureus* ability to induce platelet activation, Kerrigan et al. perfused platelets over an immobilised monolayer of S. *aureus* in a parallel flow chamber. This method demonstrated that platelets perfused over S. *aureus* under shear conditions equivalent to arterial pressure led to very strong adhesion followed by rapid aggregate formation (Kerrigan et al., 2008). Deletion of ClfA from S. *aureus,* abolished adhesion and aggregate formation under all shear rates investigated. Using a plasma-free system, fibrinogen led to single platelet adhesion but not aggregate formation. Specific immunoglobulin failed to have any effect on either platelet adhesion or aggregation. However, addition of fibrinogen and specific immunoglobulin to the plasma-free system led to platelet adhesion followed by aggregate formation (Kerrigan et al., 2008) thus highlighting the importance of fibrinogen and IgG in aggregate formation induced by *S. aureus*. No interaction was seen under low shear conditions using a parallel flow chamber.

S. aureus have a wide array of proteins expressed on their surface. This protein expression profile is most likely part of their survival. For example, ClfA is expressed weakly at the exponential phase of growth whereas is expressed strongly at the stationary phase of growth. In contrast to this another major *S. aureus* protein, fibronectin binding protein A (FnBPA) is strongly expressed at the exponential phase of growth and weakly expressed at the stationary phase of growth.

FnBPA is a 112kDa cell wall bound protein which binds plasma fibronectin and immunoglobulin. Fnbp contain a specific immunoglobulin binding domain (A domain) and a separate fibronectin binding domain (BCD). The FnBPA A domain is similar in structure and function to that of the ClfA A domain. FnBPA possesses two different but related mechanisms of engaging and activating platelets (Fitzgerald et al., 2006b). In the first mechanism, fibrinogen can bind to the A domain which crosslinks to GPIIb/IIIa, and specific immunoglobulin must crosslink to FcγRIIa to trigger platelet activation and aggregation (Fitzgerald et al., 2006b). In the second mechanism the fibronectin binding domain, BCD, can independently activate platelets. Fibronectin can bind to *S. aureus* via the FnBPA BCD domain by the tandem β-zipper mechanism (Meenan et al., 2007; Raibaud et al., 2005; Schwarz et al., 2003) and also to platelet GPIIbIIIa through the common integrin recognition motif RGD (Fitzgerald et al., 2006b). The signal to trigger platelet activation/aggregation is complete when specific immunoglobulin binds the A domain of FnBPA and cross links to platelet FcγRIIa.

Clumping factor B is a 98 kDa protein highly expressed on the surface of *S. aureus* during the exponential phase of growth and shares sequence homology with ClfA (McAleese et al., 2001). Similar to ClfA, ClfB can also bind fibrinogen and specific immunoglobulin. Deletion of the fibrinogen binding site on ClfB led to a slower aggregation. Characterization of this slower response suggested that complement assembly was required along with immunoglobulin to trigger aggregation (Miajlovic et al., 2007). Therefore similar to *S. aureus* ClfA and FnBPA, ClfB is also capable of triggering platelet aggregation via 2 specific mechanisms; fibrinogen and immunoglobulin or complement and immunoglobulin. Although the complement receptor on platelets has not yet been definitively identified in these interactions, Nguyen et al. has demonstrated that *S. aureus* protein A is capable of binding to the complement receptor gC1qR/p33 (Nguyen et al., 2000). As gC1qR/p33 is only expressed on platelets upon activation rather than at resting, it suggests that the complement interaction may act as an anchor, as it this interaction occurs after the initial platelet activation response.

Staphylococcal protein A (SpA) is a 55kDa protein expressed on greater than 90% of *S. aureus* strains. SpA is made up of 5 repeat domains (A-E) which have been shown to bind to the A1 domain of the major plasma protein vonWillebrand factor with high affinity (low nM range) (Hartleib et al., 2000; O'Seaghdha et al., 2006). Platelets express a high affinity vonWillebrand factor receptor called GPIbα (Andrews et al., 2003). Under very high shear conditions, Pawar and colleagues demonstrated that deletion of SpA from *S. aureus* significantly reduced its interaction with platelets (Pawar et al., 2004). Furthermore, preincubating platelet rich plasma with a vonWillebrand Factor antibody or indeed blocking the platelet GPIbα receptor with an inhibitory monoclonal antibody partially inhibited the platelet-*S. aureus* interaction (Pawar et al., 2004). Thus highlighting the importance of this platelet specific receptor in recognising *S. aureus*.

Bacteria	Bacterial protein	Platelet receptor	Bridging protein	Response
Staphylococcus aureus	α-toxin	None	None	Aggregation
	Lipoteichoic acid	Not identified	None	Aggregation
	Protein A	FcγRIIa, gC1R/p33, GPIbα	IgG, complement, vonWillebrand factor	Aggregation / adhesion / thrombus formation
	ClfA	GPIIbIIIa, FcγRIIa,	Fibrinogen, IgG & complement	Aggregation / thrombus formation
	SdrC	Not identified	Not identified	Thrombus formation
	SdrD	Not identified	Not identified	Thrombus formation
	SdrE	Not identified	Not identified	Thrombus formation
	FnbpA/B	GPIIbIIIa, FcγRIIa	Fibrinogen, IgG & complement	Aggregation / thrombus formation
	ClfB	GPIIbIIIa, FcγRIIa	Fibrinogen, IgG & complement	
	SraP	Not identified	None	Thrombus formation
	IsdB	GPIIbIIIa	None	Aggregation / adhesion

Table 1. List of molecular interactions between Staphylococci and platelets that contribute to Infective Endocarditis

Serine rich protein SraP is a 227kDa large protein and a member of the highly conserved family of serine rich surface glycoproteins expressed on the cell wall of *S. aureus* (Siboo et al., 2005). A mutant strain of *S. aureus* lacking expression of SraP displayed signs of reduced virulence in a rabbit model of infective endocarditis, implicating its role in the development of a growing thrombus on a cardiac valve. The platelet receptor that SraP binds to is not currently known. SraP shares similarility with a group of cell wall-associated glycoproteins (Ramboarina et al., 2010) found in a number of other organisms including *Streptococcus sanguinis* (Plummer et al., 2005), *Streptococcus gordonii* (Kerrigan et al., 2007) both of which have been have been shown to bind to platelet GPIbα. Interestingly however, SraP does not seem to bind to GPIbα.

In vivo, *S. aureus* has restricted access to iron and as a result express iron regulated surface proteins to capture haem from haemogloblin and transport it into the cell (Skaar and Schneewind, 2004). Iron-regulated surface determinant B (IsdB) is a 70kDa family member that has been shown to bind to the platelet fibrinogen receptor GPIIbIIIa. *S. aureus* grown in iron limited conditions bound to platelets in a plasma free environment, suggesting that a plasma bridge bridge is not necessary for interacting with or inducing platelet activation. Mutants defective in the expression of IsdB were unable to adhere to or aggregate platelets. Using surface plasmon resonance Miajlovic et al demonstrated a direct interaction between purified GPIIbIIIa and recombinant IsdB (Miajlovic et al., 2010).

In addition to *S. aureus* having the ability to interact with platelet either directly or indirectly Youssefian and colleagues reported that platelets were also capable of internalising *S. aureus* (Youssefian et al., 2002). While internalisation corresponded with platelet activation the mechanism through which this occurred is currently not known. Moreover it is also yet to be established whether the *S. aureus* is destroyed once internalised in a manner similar to phagocytosis by immune cells.

7. Platelet-bacterial interactions: The Streptococcus

Viridans streptococci are common commensals of the oral cavity, respiratory tract, and gastrointestinal mucosa. In their respective environment these microorganisms are harmless, however following trauma to the mucous membranes they can enter to the normally sterile environment of the bloodstream. Once inside the bloodstream the viridans streptococci act as pathogens (Baddour et al., 1989) and often colonise heart valves, causing infective endocarditis (Moreillon et al., 2002) or become implanted in atherosclerotic plaques, exacerbating atherosclerosis (Chiu, 1999) mainly through an interaction with platelets (Table 2).

Streptococcus sanguinis is a common oral microorganism that is isolated from patients with infective endocarditis. In fact early studies demonstrated that 60% of *S. sanguinis* strains induced platelet aggregation in vitro (Herzberg and Meyer, 1996). Douglas et al provided strong evidence that there is a relationship between the virulence of the infecting *S. sanguinis* strains and their ability to aggregate platelets *in vitro (Douglas et al., 1990). S. sanguinis* induced platelet aggregation was largely found to be dependent on physiological concentrations of calcium and fibrinogen, and some strains required non-specific antibody. Platelet adhesion to *S. sanguinis* occurred independently of calcium, fibrinogen or non-specific antibody, suggesting that platelet adhesion and platelet aggregation are mediated independently of each other (Kerrigan et al., 2002). These observations led to the early model of platelet bacterial interaction where a class I component mediated adhesion to the platelet, a class II component mediates a calcium dependent activation of the platelet and finally a class III component mediates a calcium and fibrinogen-dependent amplification of the response (Herzberg, 1996).

The initial studies focused on identifying the class I and class II components. Treatment of *S. sanguinis* with L- (tosylamido-2-phenyl) ethyl chloromethyl ketone (TPCK)-trypsin liberated cell free peptides (Herzberg et al., 1983). Purification of these peptides failed to support platelet adhesion or trigger platelet aggregation, however, did inhibit *S. sanguinis* mediated platelet aggregation and adhesion. This studies concluded that that these TPCK-tryptic peptides contained antigenic determinants that recognise platelets thus preventing *S.*

sanguinis from binding. Using immunoaffinity chromatography and ion exchange chromatography, Erickson and colleagues identified a platelet aggregation-associated protein (PAAP) (Erickson and Herzberg, 1990). PAAP is synthesized as a 150 kDa glycoprotein which is 40% carbohydrate and is constitutively expressed on the surface of *S. sanguinis* (Erickson and Herzberg, 1993; Erickson et al., 1992). The peptide sequence pro-gly-glu-gln-gly-pro-lys in the PAAP conforms to a predicted consensus motif common to the platelet interactive domain of collagen, lys-pro-gly-glu-pro-gly-pro-lys (Erickson and Herzberg, 1990). More recently Herzberg and colleagues identified a putative collagen-binding protein containing 2 PAAP sequences (Herzberg et al., 2005). PAAP is environmentally controlled during infection in response to high temperature (fever) or exposed collagen (exposed on damaged blood vessels or damaged heart valves) (Heimdahl et al., 1990). Partial sequence alignment shows homology of PAAP to heat shock proteins of *Mycobacterium tuberculosis* and *E. coli* (Herzberg and Meyer, 1996). The platelet receptor for PAAP is currently unidentified.

Ford et al demonstrated that *S. sanguinis* strain NCTC 7863 induced aggregation of normal platelets suspended in plasma however removal of plasma proteins abolished platelet aggregation (Ford et al., 1996). The long lag time (12-15mins) of *S. sanguinis* strain 7863 was progressively shortened by incubating the bacteria in plasma for increasing lengths of time prior to addition to platelets. This suggested that plasma proteins were essential for platelet aggregation. Subsequent experiments demonstrated that complement assembly on the surface of the bacteria was necessary for aggregation of platelets. Further experiments demonstrated that complement assembly was not enough to trigger platelet aggregation which led to the discovery that IgG and fibrinogen was necessary to complete the aggregation process (Ford et al., 1997). More recently McNicol and colleagues demonstrated that depletion of *S. sanguinis*-specific antibodies from plasma prevented platelet aggregation (McNicol et al., 2006). Following *S. sanguinis* binding, addition of antibodies led to rapid phosphorylation of the platelet antibody receptor, FcγRIIa (Pampolina and McNicol, 2005) and further downstream effector targets such as phospholipase Cγ2, syk and adapter molecule LAT.

In 2002 Kerrigan et al, demonstrated that *S. sanguinis* strain 133-79 bound to the platelet vonWillebrand factor receptor, GPIbα (Kerrigan et al., 2002). There was no requirement for vonWillebrand factor or immunoglobulin binding in this system, suggesting that *S. sanguinis* binds directly to platelet GPIbα. Confirmation for the role of GPIbα was provided when a range of site-specific inhibitory monoclonal antibodies against GPIbα prevented *S. sanguis* binding to the platelet. In addition, enzymatic cleavage of GPIbα using the snake venom from a viper pit localised the binding region within the N-terminal 1-225 portion of GPIbα. Finally, platelets from patients with Bernard Soulier Syndrome (patients who fail to express GPIbα on the surface of their platelets) did not aggregate in response to *S. sanguinis* (Kerrigan et al., 2002). The *S. sanguinis* protein that binds GPIbα was purified from cell wall extracts by chromatography on GPIbα and wheat germ agglutinin affinity matrices (Plummer et al., 2005). This led to the identification of a highly glycosylated serine-rich protein called serine-rich protein A (SrpA). An insertional inactivation mutant lacking the SrpA of *S. sanguinis* showed a significant increase in the lag time to aggregation, implicating this protein in platelet aggregation. In addition, platelet adhesion to the SrpA mutant was significantly reduced, however not abolished, suggesting other factors are involved in supporting platelet adhesion.

Streptococcus gordonii is a close but distinct relative of *S. sanguinis* (Nobbs et al., 2009), however initial reports suggested that *S. gordonii* could not induce platelet aggregation (Douglas et al., 1990). More in depth characterisation has demonstrated that *S. gordonii* is capable of supporting platelet adhesion and inducing platelets aggregation in a strain dependent manner. Glycosylated surface protein B is a large 280kDa protein expressed on the surface of *S. gordonii* strain M99. It is heavily glycosylated with glucose and glucosamine and is transported to the cell surface via an accessory system compromising of the SecA2 and the SecY2 proteins (Bensing and Sullam, 2002; Takahashi et al., 2004). GspB has been shown to be highly homologous to an expanding family of Gram-positive bacterial cell surface proteins that includes *S. aureus* serine rich protein SraP (Siboo et al., 2005) *S. sanguis* serine-rich protein SrpA (Plummer et al., 2005), *S. gordonii* DL1 sialic acid-binding protein Hsa (Takahashi et al., 2002) and the *S. parasanguinis* fimbriae-associated protein Fap1 (Wu et al., 2007). These proteins were originally discovered because of their ability to bind a variety of sialylated glycoproteins. Platelet GPIbα is an example of a sialylated glycoprotein and as a result has been shown to bind *S. gordonii* GspB and Hsa (Bensing et al., 2004). Additional molecular glycan characterisation demonstrated that GspB specifically binds O-linked sialic acid residues on GPIbα (Takamatsu et al., 2005), whereas Hsa specifically binds N-linked sialic acid residues on GPIbα and GPIIbIIIa (Yajima et al., 2005). Interestingly an isogenic mutant lacking the expression of Hsa in *S. gordonii* strain DL1 failed to affect percent platelet aggregation however reduced platelet adhesion by ~ 50%. These more recent functional studies suggest that additional protein interactions are necessary for supporting platelet adhesion (Jakubovics et al., 2005a).

S. gordonii expresses a large protein of ~3500 amino acids with a high molecular weight of 397 kDa designated platelet adherence protein A (PadA) (Petersen et al., 2010). PadA contains a short stretch of amino acid residues which displays weak homology to A1 and C1 domain of the plasma protein, vonWillebrand factor (vWf). These domains in vWf are essential for interactions with platelet GPIb and GPIIb/IIIa, respectively. Disruption of the PadA gene from *S. gordonii* DL1 failed to affect binding to glycocalacin (soluble purified GPIbα), however, ablated binding to purified GPIIb/IIIa. Furthermore, platelet adhesion to *S. gordonii* DL1 was significantly reduced by preincubation of platelets with an integrin recognition RGD-containing peptide or the GPIIb/IIIa inhibitor, abciximab (Petersen et al., 2010). Earlier studies demonstrated that *S. gordonii* DL1 bound specifically to GPIIb but not GPIIIa of the GPIIbIIIa complex (Yajima et al., 2005). Collectively these results suggest that platelet adhesion is a mutlifactorial event where Hsa binds GPIbα and PadA binds GPIIb/IIIa and together they act synergistically to support platelet adhesion.

Platelets are very sensitive to shear and some platelet-substrate interactions only manifest themselves upon exposure to shear. For example, under low shear conditions there is no interaction between platelets and vWf however under high shear conditions platelets roll along the vWf coated surface (Ruggeri, 2009). Perfusing platelets over immobilised *S. sanguinis* or *S. gordonii* in a parallel flow chamber under low shear (veneous shear), platelets interacted with a typical rolling behaviour followed by firm adhesion (Jakubovics et al., 2005a; Plummer et al., 2005). This phenomena is highly characteristic of platelet rolling on damaged endothelium (Ruggeri, 2009). Rolling is mediated by platelet GPIbα where is the fast on-off rate of the receptor allows loss of interaction between GPIbα and the bacteria on one side of the platelet leading to the formation of another GPIbα-bacterial interaction on the other side of the platelet. Deletion of the *S. sanguinis* GPIbα-binding protein SrpA or indeed the *S. gordonii* GPIbα-binding protein Hsa abolished the rolling behaviour, suggesting that these proteins form the initial attachment of platelets with the bacteria under physiological shear conditions. Soluble vWf exists in the plasma in a conformation that is not recognisable by platelet GPIbα. However at the site of injury, vWf binds to extracellular matrix proteins forming a thrombotic surface for the platelet. Typically platelets roll along immobilised vWf under high shear conditions. The high shear induces a conformational change in vWf making it recognisable to GPIbα. As *S. gordonii* Hsa and *S. sanguis* SrpA can support static platelet adhesion, or indeed mediate rolling of platelets under low shear conditions it suggests that Hsa and SrpA exist in a unique conformation that is recognisable by GPIbα, as their receptor conformation is not believed to be altered when subjected to shear. The process of rolling is to slow the platelet down from the high shear force experienced in the vasculature long enough to allow it firmly adhere to the bacteria. Firm adhesion is complete when platelet GPIIb/IIIa interacts with *S. gordonii* PadA.

Once the platelets become firmly adhered to *S. gordonii* by engaging with either GPIbα or GPIIbIIIa, a signal is generated in the platelet that results in the platelet changing shape and spreading out on the bacterial surface. The function of platelet spreading is essential for the platelet to withstand the shear forces experienced in the vasculature. Platelet spreading is a particularly important in the development of thrombotic vegetations in infective endocarditis because the lesions around the lesion on the cardiac valve are often very turbulent. Therefore, platelets require the conversion from a discoid shape to a fully spread cell to withstand turbulent shear force. Keane et al, demonstrated that engagement of either GPIbα or GPIIbIIIa, the ITAM-bearing receptor, FcγRIIa and its downstream effectors syk and phospholipase Cγ2 became tyrosine phosphorylated which suggests that this pathway is essential for platelet spreading (Keane et al., 2010a). In addition tyrosine phosphorylation of the FcγRIIa resulted in platelet degranulation, a step critical for inducing and amplyfing platelet aggregation.

Once platelets become firmly adhered and a signal is generated in the platelet it leads to platelet aggregation. Interestingly, while a mutant *S. gordonii* strain lacking expression of Hsa displayed reduced ability to support platelet adhesion, platelet aggregation remained unaffected. This observation suggests that different proteins expressed on the surface of *S. gordonii* mediate different interactions and subsequent responses in platelets. To address this Kerrigan et al used a proteomic approach to identify differentially expressed proteins on a strain of *S. gordonii* that induces platelet aggregation (*S. gordonii* strain DL1) versus one that does not (*S. gordonii* strain Blackburn). Cell wall proteins from both strains were removed from the cell wall using lysozyme. Recovered proteins were separated by poly-acrylamide gel electrophoresis and 2 bands corresponding to 172 kDa and 164 kDa were shown to be differentially expressed. Mass spectrometry identified these proteins as antigen I/II (Kerrigan et al., 2007). The antigen I/II family of proteins are probably the best characterised proteins on the surface of *S. gordonii*. Originally identified on *Streptococcus mutans*, antigen I/II have now been identified on almost all oral streptococci (Nobbs et al., 2007). In *S. gordonii*, antigen I/II have been designated SspA/B. These proteins are oligospecific adhesins which have been shown to bind to several ligands such as collagen type I (Heddle et al., 2003), β_1 integrins (Nobbs et al., 2007), salivary agglutinin glycoprotein (Prakobphol et al., 2000) as well as other bacteria including *P. gingivalis*, *Candida albicans* and *Actinomyces naeslundii* (Demuth et al., 2001; Egland et al., 2001; Jakubovics et al., 2005b). Deletion of SspA/B from *S. gordonii* DL1 failed to affect either platelet aggregation or platelet adhesion. However, deletion of SspA/B and Hsa together abolished platelet aggregation and reduced platelet adhesion by 50%, similar to the Hsa mutant alone (Kerrigan et al., 2007). Consistent with this over expression of SspA and SspB in the non-platelet reactive surrogate host *Lactococcus lactis* induced platelet aggregation but failed to support platelet adhesion. These results suggest that SspA/B and Hsa must act synergistically when binding to platelets to trigger aggregation and that they are not involved in supporting platelet adhesion. At present the receptor through which SspA/B binds to on the platelets is not current known.

Bacteria	Bacterial protein	Platelet receptor	Bridging protein	Response
S. sanguinis	PAAP	Not identified	None	Aggregation
	Not identified	FcγRIIa	Antibody, fibrinogen & complement	Aggregation
	SrpA	GPIbα	None	Adhesion / aggregation
S. gordonii	GspB	GPIbα	None	Adhesion
	Hsa	GPIbα	None	Adhesion / aggregation
	PadA	GPIIbIIIa	None	Adhesion
	SspA/B	Not identified	None	Adhesion / Aggregation
S. mitis	PblA/B	Not identified	None	Aggregation
	Lysin	GPIIbIIIa	fibrinogen	Aggregation
S. mutans	Rgp	Not identified	IgG	Aggregation
	PAc	Not identified	None	Aggregation
S. oralis	Not identified	Not identified	None	Adhesion / aggregation
S. parasanguinis	FimA	Not identified	None	?
	Fap1	Not identified	None	Adhesion
S. pneumoniae	Not identified	TLR2	None	Aggregation

Table 2. List of molecular interactions between Streptococci and platelets that contribute to Infective Endocarditis

Streptococcus mitis has also been shown to interact with platelets although reports are conflicting. In 1990, Douglas et al, used several strains of *S. mitis* and found that none of these interacted with platelets. Ohkuni and colleagues suggested that *S. mitis* strain Nm-65

released a 66 kDa protein (*S.mitis*-derived human platelet aggregation factor, Sm-PAF) that induced platelet aggregation (Ohkuni et al., 1997). Characterisation of this secreted protein revealed that it was a toxin that lysed platelets rather than induced platelet aggregation. More recent work by Bensing et al, identified two distinct genetic loci of *S. mitis* strain SF100 that contributes to platelet binding (Bensing et al., 2001a). The first locus encodes PblT. The mechanism through which it binds to platelets has not yet been explored. The second locus encodes two cell wall associated proteins; PblA is a 107 kDa protein and PblB which is a 121 kDa protein (Bensing et al., 2001b). These proteins are unique as neither of the proteins expresses homology to any other bacterial adhesins described, however share similarities with structural components of bacteriophages (Mitchell et al., 2007). Bacteria often bind to oligosaccharides on host cells. For example *S. gordonii* GspB binds to α2-3-linked sialic acids on platelets and salivary mucins. Platelets treated with sialidases having different linkage specificities demonstrated that removal of α2-8-linked sialic acids resulted in a reduction in *S. mitis* SF100 binding. Gangliosides are glycosphingolipids rich in sialic acids and are found in abundance in lipid rafts in platelets (Marcus et al., 1972). *S. mitis* strains lacking the expression of PblA and PblB demonstrated significant decrease in platelet binding invitro as well as marked reduction in virulence in an animal model of infective endocarditis (Bensing et al., 2001b; Mitchell et al., 2007). More recent studies have demonstrated that *S. mitis* surface bound lysin can bind both free and platelet bound fibrinogen, through its interaction with the Aa and Bb chains of fibrinogen (Seo et al., 2010). Once *S. mitis* has bound fibrinogen this in turn can bind to the platelet fibrinogen receptor, GPIIbIIIa, initiating thrombus formation.

Although early reports suggest *Streptococcus oralis* is capable of inducing platelet aggregation and supporting platelet adhesion the exact mechanism through which either of these occur is currently unknown.

Streptococcus mutans strain Xc induces platelet aggregation by releasing extracts containing serotype-specific polysaccharides which are composed of rhamnose-glucose polymers. An isogenic mutant lacking synthesis the rhamnose-glucose polymers significantly reduced platelet aggregation (Chia et al., 2004). *S. mutans* failed to induce platelet aggregation in the absence of plasma proteins suggesting that a plasma protein possibly bridges the bacteria to the platelet. Subsequent studies identified that addition of serotype-specific IgG to plasma free platelets restored aggregation. The ability of rhamnose polymers toinduce platelet aggregation has been known for some time. For example, ristocetin is obtained from Amycolatopsis lurida and is well characterised for its ability to induce platelet agglutination. The mechanism of ristocetin induced agglutination of platelets involves vWf binding to platelet GPIbα. Cleavage of the rhamnose tetrasaccharide of ristocetin abolished its ability to induce platelet aggregation (Bardsley et al., 1998). Moreover, *S. sanguinis* expresses a platelet associated aggregating protein (PAAP) which is another rhamnose polymer which is thought to be involved in inducing platelet aggregation. Together these results suggest that rhamnose plays an important role in inducing platelet aggregation. Additional studies by Munro et al, demonstrated that an isogenic mutant of *S. mutans* strain V403 lacking the exopolysaccharides glucan and fructan had decreased infectivity in the rat model of endocarditis compared to the wild-type strain (Munro and Macrina, 1993). Protein antigen C (PAc) is a high molecular weight protein expressed by *S. mutans* that has been shown to interact with an unidentified platelet protein (Matsumoto-Nakano et al., 2009). Clinical strains that do not naturally express PAc failed to induce platelet aggregation.

Although the platelet receptor that recognises PAc was not identified, the authors demonstrated that increasing amounts of anti-PAc serum significantly reduced platelet aggregation, suggesting that antibody recognition may be a critical factor.

Streptococcus parasanguinis expresses a 36kDa surface protein called FimA. A mutant defective on the expression of FimA from *S. parasanguinis* strain FW213 failed to have any effect on supporting platelet adhesion or inducing platelet aggregation however significantly reduced the extent of endocarditis in the rat model (Burnette-Curley et al., 1995). Based on these observations the exact mechanism by which FimA functions as a virulence factor of endocarditis has yet to be determined, however it is possible that FimA plays a role in adherence to fibrin deposits associated with damaged heart valves. Fimbrae-associated protein 1 (Fap1) is a highly glycosylated serine-rich glycoprotein which shares sequence and structural homology with SrpA of *S. sanguinis*, GspB of *S. gordonii* and SraP of *S. aureus*. SrpA of *S. sanguinis* and GspB of *S. gordonii* have both been shown to interact directly with platelet GPIbα to trigger platelet activation (Wu et al., 2007). To date no studies have demonstrated that Fap1 interacts with GPIbα or indeed with platelets directly.

Early studies by Johnson et al, demonstrated that at low concentrations *Streptococcus pneumoniae* pneumolysin had little effect on platelets, however at higher concentrations platelets were lysed presumably by binding to the sterols present in the platelet plasma membrane and forming multimeric transmembrane pores (Johnson et al., 1981). The ability to form these pores may result in lysis of platelets. Lysis occurred in a time-dependent manner where greater than 50% of platelets were lysed. A more recent study demonstrated that a concentrated sample of supernatant from an overnight growth of *S. pneumoniae* that contained pneumolysin failed to induce human platelet aggregation, moreover a pneumolysin-negative strain of *S. pneumoniae* also induced platelet aggregation suggesting that pneumolysin is not involved in inducing platelet aggregation (Keane et al., 2010b). In this report the authors demonstrated that *S. pneumoniae* binds to platelet toll like receptor 2 (TLR2), a pattern recognition receptor which triggered the PI3kinase/RAP1 pathway which leads to activation of the fibrinogen receptor GPIIbIIIa.

8. Platelet-bacterial interactions: Non staphylococcal, non streptococcal

There is no doubt Staphylococcus and Streptococcus species make up the majority of cases of infective endocarditis, however other opportunistic pathogens, while rare, may also play a role (Table 3). For example recent work by Shannon et al. demonstrated that clinical isolates of *Enterococcus faecalis* induced platelet aggregation. The ability of the *E. faecalis* to induce platelet aggregation was dependent on IgG (Rasmussen et al., 2010). *Helicobacter pylori* has also been shown to interact with platelets. When in plasma it binds vonWillebrand factor, which in turn enables it to interact with GPIbα and trigger platelet aggregation. This is a unique interaction as soluble vonWillebrand factor cannot interact with platelet GPIbα. The *H. pylori* protein that binds vonWillebrand factor is currently not identified (Byrne et al., 2003; Corcoran et al., 2007). *Porphyromonas ginigvalis* secretes a protease called gingipains that acts directly on platelet protease activated receptors (Lourbakos et al., 2001). Naito and colleagues also deomstrated that *P. ginigvalis* expresses a protein called Hgp44 which also induces platelet aggregation. Although the platelet receptor has not been definitively identified antibodies against GPIbα abolish the interaction (Naito et al., 2006). Finally, *Escherichia coli* secretes shiga-like toxin which binds to the glycosphingolipid receptors on the surface of the platelet and triggers platelet activation (Cooling et al., 1998), however other groups failed to see the interaction in vivo (Viisoreanu et al., 2000). One explanation for these contradictory results is that in vivo the actions of Shiga toxins are complex and many of its actions on platelets are indirect being mediated through effects on other cells such as monocytes (Guessous et al., 2005) and endothelial cells (Motto et al., 2005).

Bacteria	Bacterial protein	Platelet receptor	Bridging protein	Response
Enterococcus faecalis	Not identified	FcgRIIa	IgG	Aggregation
Helicobacter pylori	Not identified	GPIbα	vonWillebrand Factor	Aggregation
Porphyromonas gingivalis	RgpA/B	PAR1 & PAR4	None	Aggregation
	Hgp44	GPIbα	Not identified	Aggregation
Escherichia coli	Shiga-like toxin	Sphingolipids	None	Aggregation

Table 3. List of molecular interactions between non staphylococcal non streptococcal microorganisms and platelets that may contribute to Infective Endocarditis

9. Current and novel treatment options for infective endocarditis

As infective endocarditis is primarily a bacteria infection, often associated with dental and other medical procedures, prophylactic antibiotic treatment was considered to be normal practice. However, more recently the American Heart Association (AHA) and American College of Cardiology (ACC) released a guidance document on infective endocarditis that significantly changed routine practice (Nishimura et al., 2008). In particular they no longer recommend the prophylactic use of antibiotics for dental or other procedures except for a small group of high-risk patients. This was primarily due to the fact that the risks associated with prophylaxis outweigh the benefits. The review panel felt that the biggest risk for IE is not dental or other procedures but rather bleeding from gums due to poor oral hygiene. Thus, so few cases of IE will be prevented by antibiotic prophylaxis during medical procedures but there will be an increase in antibiotic resistance that the there is little benefit to prophylaxis. They felt that improved oral hygiene would be more effective at preventing the occurrence of IE. The exception was for very high-risk patients, which are basically patients with prosthetic valves or those with a history of IE.

With the increase in antibiotic-resistant strains of pathogenic bacteria researchers have been looking at new strategies to target bacteria. One such approach is to target the host response to the pathogen (Clatworthy et al., 2007). IE is very amenable to this strategy as it basically arises from an ineffective host response to the infection. If the platelet aggregation response can be prevented there would be no thrombus formation.

The obvious strategy would be to use an anti-platelet agent to prevent the thrombus formation. Aspirin is the most widely used anti-platelet agent and acts to inhibit cyclooxygenase but may not be effective in preventing IE (Chan et al., 2003). While aspirin effectively inhibits COX some bacteria can activate platelets in a COX-independent manner. As it is not known prior to the procedure which bacteria are likely to be involved aspirin would not be sufficient. A more effective strategy would be to use a $P2Y_{12}$ antagonist such as clopidogrel. However, its very effectiveness makes it unlikely to be used. The inhibition of platelet function by clopidogrel and other anti-platelet agents cause bleeding and it is unlikely that dentists would be happy to perform extractions and other such procedures when the patient is likely to experience very heavy bleeding. Certainly surgeons will not operate on a patient on clopidogrel and they typically require a reversal of the inhibition before they will consider surgery.

Targeting the bacteria is an approach that is attractive, as it would not interfere with platelet function. However, as we have seen choosing a target is difficult as every species of bacteria interact differently with platelets and even different strains of the same species can interact differently (Fitzgerald et al., 2006a). There is also the problem that bacteria such as *S. aureus* have multiple interactions with platelets and it is not clear which one if any is the critical one during IE. Certainly if it was possible to identify a single bacterial protein that was conserved across many pathogenic strains and was found to be critical in the interaction with platelets it would be possible to produce a vaccine against it (Broughan et al., 2011).

Despite the limitations associated with the use of anti-platelet agents platelets are still a promising target for any potential new drug. This is because so far there are only a few platelet receptors implicated in the response to bacteria primarily GPIIb/IIIa and GPIbα. GPIIb/IIIa plays an important role in *S. aureus*-and *S. gordonii* mediated platelet aggregation but as the fibrinogen receptor it also plays a critical role in platelet aggregation. Because of this important role in platelet function a number of inhibitors of this receptor have been developed. Although only for intravenous use these drugs have been very effective anti-platelet agents (Curtin, 2004). However, they are very potent in their inhibition and will cause a profound inhibition of platelet function along with a prolongation of bleeding time that will not be suitable for prophylaxis during procedures such as dental manipulations.

A second platelet receptor that is important in the platelet response to bacteria is GPIbα, which is the von Willebrand factor receptor. GPIbα is very important in platelet adhesion under shear stress and is a very attractive target in cardiovascular disease. However, despite the efforts of many researchers to discover GPIbα inhibitors none have yet made it to the market (Vanhoorelbeke et al., 2007).

FcγRIIa has been shown to mediate platelet activation by many different bacteria including Staphylococci and Streptococci. It typically acts in conjunction with GPIbα, GPIIb/IIIa or the complement receptor. Unlike receptors such as GPIbα and GPIIb/IIIa FcγRIIa is not involved in thrombosis as its role are primarily involved in the immune function of platelets. Thus, antagonists of FcγRIIa will have little impact on platelet function and will not cause bleeding problems making it an ideal target for prophylactic therapy for IE.

The interaction between platelets and bacteria is the key element of infective endocarditis. While there are many different bacterial proteins that can bind to platelets there are only a few potential receptors on the platelet for these proteins. This makes the platelet a good target for novel strategies to inhibit this interaction. While there is always a risk of causing bleeding problems with anti-platelet agents FcγRIIa has been found to be the critical receptor on platelets for the interaction with bacteria. As this receptor is associated with the innate immune functions of platelets rather than with its role in thrombosis targeting FcγRIIa will have minimal effects on the role of platelets in thrombosis. This strategy would be in line with the recent guidance document on infective endocarditis from AHA/ACC. Prophylactic use of an FcγRIIa antagonist during medical procedures with no risk of developing resistance. Antibiotic therapy could then be reserved for cases of sepsis or confirmed infective endocarditis.

10. References

Andrews, R.K., E.E. Gardiner, Y. Shen, J.C. Whisstock, and M.C. Berndt. 2003. Glycoprotein Ib-IX-V. *Int J Biochem Cell Biol* 35:1170-1174.

Antczak, A.J., N. Singh, S.R. Gay, and R.G. Worth. 2010. IgG-complex stimulated platelets: A source of sCD40L and RANTES in initiation of inflammatory cascade. *Cellular Immunology* 263:129-133.

Arvand, M., S. Bhakdi, B. Dahlback, and K.T. Preissner. 1990. Staphylococcus aureus alpha-toxin attack on human platelets promotes assembly of the prothrombinase complex. *J Biol Chem* 265:14377-14381.

Asopa, S., A. Patel, O.A. Khan, R. Sharma, and S.K. Ohri. 2007. Non-bacterial thrombotic endocarditis. *Eur J Cardiothorac Surg* 32:696-701.

Baddour, L.M., G.D. Christensen, J.H. Lowrance, and W.A. Simpson. 1989. Pathogenesis of experimental endocarditis. *Rev Infect Dis* 11:452-463.

Baddour, L.M., W.R. Wilson, A.S. Bayer, V.G. Fowler, Jr., A.F. Bolger, M.E. Levison, P. Ferrieri, M.A. Gerber, L.Y. Tani, M.H. Gewitz, D.C. Tong, J.M. Steckelberg, R.S. Baltimore, S.T. Shulman, J.C. Burns, D.A. Falace, J.W. Newburger, T.J. Pallasch, M. Takahashi, and K.A. Taubert. 2005. Infective Endocarditis: Diagnosis, Antimicrobial Therapy, and Management of Complications: A Statement for Healthcare Professionals From the Committee on Rheumatic Fever, Endocarditis, and Kawasaki Disease, Council on Cardiovascular Disease in the Young, and the Councils on Clinical Cardiology, Stroke, and Cardiovascular Surgery and Anesthesia, American Heart Association: Endorsed by the Infectious Diseases Society of America. *Circulation* 111:e394-434.

Baliakina, E.V., E.V. Gerasimovskaia, A. Romanov Iu, and E. Atakhanov Sh. 1999. [Role of staphylococcus aureus hemolytic toxin-alpha in pathogenesis of infectious endocarditis: studies in vitro]. *Ter Arkh* 71:28-31.

Bardsley, B., D.H. Williams, and T.P. Baglin. 1998. Cleavage of rhamnose from ristocetin A removes its ability to induce platelet aggregation. *Blood Coagul Fibrinolysis* 9:241-244.

Bayer, A.S., D. Cheng, M.R. Yeaman, G.R. Corey, R.S. McClelland, L.J. Harrel, and V.G. Fowler, Jr. 1998. In vitro resistance to thrombin-induced platelet microbicidal protein among clinical bacteremic isolates of Staphylococcus aureus correlates with an endovascular infectious source. *Antimicrob Agents Chemother* 42:3169-3172.

Bayer, A.S., M.D. Ramos, B.E. Menzies, M.R. Yeaman, A.J. Shen, and A.L. Cheung. 1997. Hyperproduction of alpha-toxin by Staphylococcus aureus results in paradoxically reduced virulence in experimental endocarditis: a host defense role for platelet microbicidal proteins. *Infect Immun* 65:4652-4660.

Bensing, B.A., J.A. Lopez, and P.M. Sullam. 2004. The Streptococcus gordonii surface proteins GspB and Hsa mediate binding to sialylated carbohydrate epitopes on the platelet membrane glycoprotein Ibalpha. *Infect Immun* 72:6528-6537.

Bensing, B.A., C.E. Rubens, and P.M. Sullam. 2001a. Genetic loci of Streptococcus mitis that mediate binding to human platelets. *Infect Immun* 69:1373-1380.

Bensing, B.A., I.R. Siboo, and P.M. Sullam. 2001b. Proteins PblA and PblB of Streptococcus mitis, which promote binding to human platelets, are encoded within a lysogenic bacteriophage. *Infect Immun* 69:6186-6192.

Bensing, B.A., and P.M. Sullam. 2002. An accessory sec locus of Streptococcus gordonii is required for export of the surface protein GspB and for normal levels of binding to human platelets. *Mol Microbiol* 44:1081-1094.

Bernheimer, A.W. 1965. Staphylococcal alpha toxin. *Ann N Y Acad Sci* 128:112-123.

Bernheimer, A.W., and L.L. Schwartz. 1965. Effect of Staphylococcal and Other Bacterial Toxins on Platelets in Vitro. *J Pathol Bacteriol* 89:209-223.

Beynon, R.P., V.K. Bahl, and B.D. Prendergast. 2006. Infective endocarditis. *Br Med J* 333:334-339.

Blair, P., S. Rex, O. Vitseva, L. Beaulieu, K. Tanriverdi, S. Chakrabarti, C. Hayashi, C.A. Genco, M. Iafrati, and J.E. Freedman. 2009. Stimulation of Toll-like receptor 2 in human platelets induces a thromboinflammatory response through activation of phosphoinositide 3-kinase. *Circ Res* 104:346-354.

Broughan, J., R. Anderson, and A.S. Anderson. 2011. Strategies for and advances in the development of Staphylococcus aureus prophylactic vaccines. *Expert Review of Vaccines* 10:695-708.

Burnette-Curley, D., V. Wells, H. Viscount, C.L. Munro, J.C. Fenno, P. Fives-Taylor, and F.L. Macrina. 1995. FimA, a major virulence factor associated with Streptococcus parasanguis endocarditis. *Infect Immun* 63:4669-4674.

Byrne, M.F., S.W. Kerrigan, P.A. Corcoran, J.C. Atherton, F.E. Murray, D.J. Fitzgerald, and D.M. Cox. 2003. Helicobacter pylori binds von Willebrand factor and interacts with GPIb to induce platelet aggregation. *Gastroenterology* 124:1846-1854.

Chan, K., J. Dumesnil, B. Cujec, A. Sanfilippo, J. Jue, M. Turek, T. Robinson, D. Moher, and I.o.t.M.A.S.i.I. Endocarditis. 2003. A randomized trial of aspirin on the risk of embolic events in patients with infective endocarditis. *J Am Coll Cardiol* 42:775-780.

Chia, J.S., Y.L. Lin, H.T. Lien, and J.Y. Chen. 2004. Platelet aggregation induced by serotype polysaccharides from Streptococcus mutans. *Infect Immun* 72:2605-2617.

Chiu, B. 1999. Multiple infections in carotid atherosclerotic plaques. *Am Heart J* 138:S534-536.

Clatworthy, A.E., E. Pierson, and D.T. Hung. 2007. Targeting virulence: a new paradigm for antimicrobial therapy. *Nat Chem Biol* 3:541-548.

Cooling, L.L., K.E. Walker, T. Gille, and T.A. Koerner. 1998. Shiga toxin binds human platelets via globotriaosylceramide (Pk antigen) and a novel platelet glycosphingolipid. *Infect Immun* 66:4355-4366.

Corcoran, P.A., J.C. Atherton, S.W. Kerrigan, T. Wadstrom, F.E. Murray, R.M. Peek, D.J. Fitzgerald, D.M. Cox, and M.F. Byrne. 2007. The effect of different strains of Helicobacter pylori on platelet aggregation. *Can J Gastroenterol* 21:367-370.

Cox, D., S.W. Kerrigan, and S.P. Watson. 2011. Platelets and the innate immune system: mechanisms of bacterial-induced platelet activation. *Journal of Thrombosis and Haemostasis* 9:1097-1107.

Curtin, R. 2004. Intravenous glycoprotein IIb/IIIa antagonists: their benefits, problems and future developments. *Curr Pharm Des* 10:1577-1585.

Demuth, D.R., D.C. Irvine, J.W. Costerton, G.S. Cook, and R.J. Lamont. 2001. Discrete protein determinant directs the species-specific adherence of Porphyromonas gingivalis to oral streptococci. *Infect Immun* 69:5736-5741.

Douglas, C.W., P.R. Brown, and F.E. Preston. 1990. Platelet aggregation by oral streptococci. *FEMS Microbiol Lett* 60:63-67.

Egland, P.G., L.D. Du, and P.E. Kolenbrander. 2001. Identification of independent Streptococcus gordonii SspA and SspB functions in coaggregation with Actinomyces naeslundii. *Infect Immun* 69:7512-7516.

Erickson, P.R., and M.C. Herzberg. 1990. Purification and partial characterization of a 65-kDa platelet aggregation-associated protein antigen from the surface of Streptococcus sanguis. *J Biol Chem* 265:14080-14087.

Erickson, P.R., and M.C. Herzberg. 1993. The Streptococcus sanguis platelet aggregation-associated protein. Identification and characterization of the minimal platelet-interactive domain. *J Biol Chem* 268:1646-1649.

Erickson, P.R., M.C. Herzberg, and G. Tierney. 1992. Cross-reactive immunodeterminants on Streptococcus sanguis and collagen. Predicting a structural motif of platelet-interactive domains. *J Biol Chem* 267:10018-10023.

Fitzgerald, J.R., T.J. Foster, and D. Cox. 2006a. The interaction of bacterial pathogens with platelets. *Nat Rev Microbiol* 4:445-457.

Fitzgerald, J.R., A. Loughman, F. Keane, M. Brennan, M. Knobel, J. Higgins, L. Visai, P. Speziale, D. Cox, and T.J. Foster. 2006b. Fibronectin-binding proteins of Staphylococcus aureus mediate activation of human platelets via fibrinogen and fibronectin bridges to integrin GPIIb/IIIa and IgG binding to the FcgammaRIIa receptor. *Mol Microbiol* 59:212-230.

Ford, I., C.W. Douglas, D. Cox, D.G. Rees, J. Heath, and F.E. Preston. 1997. The role of immunoglobulin G and fibrinogen in platelet aggregation by Streptococcus sanguis. *Br J Haematol* 97:737-746.

Ford, I., C.W. Douglas, J. Heath, C. Rees, and F.E. Preston. 1996. Evidence for the involvement of complement proteins in platelet aggregation by Streptococcus sanguis NCTC 7863. *Br J Haematol* 94:729-739.

Fowler, V.G., Jr., L.M. McIntyre, M.R. Yeaman, G.E. Peterson, L. Barth Reller, G.R. Corey, D. Wray, and A.S. Bayer. 2000. In vitro resistance to thrombin-induced platelet microbicidal protein in isolates of Staphylococcus aureus from endocarditis patients correlates with an intravascular device source. *J Infect Dis* 182:1251-1254.

George, N.P., K. Konstantopoulos, and J.M. Ross. 2007. Differential kinetics and molecular recognition mechanisms involved in early versus late growth phase Staphylococcus aureus cell binding to platelet layers under physiological shear conditions. *J Infect Dis* 196:639-646.

George, N.P., Q. Wei, P.K. Shin, K. Konstantopoulos, and J.M. Ross. 2006. Staphylococcus aureus adhesion via Spa, ClfA, and SdrCDE to immobilized platelets demonstrates shear-dependent behavior. *Arterioscler Thromb Vasc Biol* 26:2394-2400.

Guessous, F., M. Marcinkiewicz, R. Polanowska-Grabowska, T.R. Keepers, T. Obrig, and A.R. Gear. 2005. Shiga toxin 2 and lipopolysaccharide cause monocytic THP-1 cells to release factors which activate platelet function. *Thromb Haemost* 94:1019-1027.

Hartleib, J., N. Kohler, R.B. Dickinson, G.S. Chhatwal, J.J. Sixma, O.M. Hartford, T.J. Foster, G. Peters, B.E. Kehrel, and M. Herrmann. 2000. Protein A is the von Willebrand factor binding protein on Staphylococcus aureus. *Blood* 96:2149-2156.

Hawiger, J., S. Steckley, D. Hammond, C. Cheng, S. Timmons, A.D. Glick, and R.M. Des Prez. 1979. Staphylococci-induced human platelet injury mediated by protein A and immunoglobulin G Fc fragment receptor. *J Clin Invest* 64:931-937.

Heddle, C., A.H. Nobbs, N.S. Jakubovics, M. Gal, J.P. Mansell, D. Dymock, and H.F. Jenkinson. 2003. Host collagen signal induces antigen I/II adhesin and invasin gene expression in oral Streptococcus gordonii. *Mol Microbiol* 50:597-607.

Heimdahl, A., G. Hall, M. Hedberg, H. Sandberg, P.O. Soder, K. Tuner, and C.E. Nord. 1990. Detection and quantitation by lysis-filtration of bacteremia after different oral surgical procedures. *J Clin Microbiol* 28:2205-2209.

Herzberg, M.C. 1996. Platelet-streptococcal interactions in endocarditis. *Crit Rev Oral Biol Med* 7:222-236.

Herzberg, M.C., K.L. Brintzenhofe, and C.C. Clawson. 1983. Cell-free released components of Streptococcus sanguis inhibit human platelet aggregation. *Infect Immun* 42:394-401.

Herzberg, M.C., and M.W. Meyer. 1996. Effects of oral flora on platelets: possible consequences in cardiovascular disease. *J Periodontol* 67:1138-1142.

Herzberg, M.C., A. Nobbs, L. Tao, A. Kilic, E. Beckman, A. Khammanivong, and Y. Zhang. 2005. Oral streptococci and cardiovascular disease: searching for the platelet aggregation-associated protein gene and mechanisms of Streptococcus sanguis-induced thrombosis. *J Periodontol* 76:2101-2105.

Hildebrand, A., M. Pohl, and S. Bhakdi. 1991. Staphylococcus aureus alpha-toxin. Dual mechanism of binding to target cells. *J Biol Chem* 266:17195-17200.

Homma, S., and C. Grahame-Clarke. 2003. Toward reducing embolic complications from endocarditis. *J Am Coll Cardiol* 42:781-783.

Ikigai, H., and T. Nakae. 1985. Conformational alteration in alpha-toxin from Staphylococcus aureus concomitant with the transformation of the water-soluble monomer to the membrane oligomer. *Biochem Biophys Res Commun* 130:175-181.

Jakubovics, N.S., S.W. Kerrigan, A.H. Nobbs, N. Stromberg, C.J. van Dolleweerd, D.M. Cox, C.G. Kelly, and H.F. Jenkinson. 2005a. Functions of cell surface-anchored antigen I/II family and Hsa polypeptides in interactions of Streptococcus gordonii with host receptors. *Infect Immun* 73:6629-6638.

Jakubovics, N.S., N. Stromberg, C.J. van Dolleweerd, C.G. Kelly, and H.F. Jenkinson. 2005b. Differential binding specificities of oral streptococcal antigen I/II family adhesins for human or bacterial ligands. *Mol Microbiol* 55:1591-1605.

Johnson, M.K., D. Boese-Marrazzo, and W A Pierce, Jr. 1981. Effects of pneumolysin on human polymorphonuclear leukocytes and platelets. *Infect Immun* 34:171-176.

Keane, C., H. Petersen, K. Reynolds, D.K. Newman, D. Cox, H.F. Jenkinson, P.J. Newman, and S.W. Kerrigan. 2010a. Mechanism of outside-in {alpha}IIb{beta}3-mediated activation of human platelets by the colonizing Bacterium, Streptococcus gordonii. *Arterioscler Thromb Vasc Biol* 30:2408-2415.

Keane, C., D. Tilley, A. Cunningham, A. Smolenski, A. Kadioglu, D. Cox, H.F. Jenkinson, and S.W. Kerrigan. 2010b. Invasive Streptococcus pneumoniae trigger platelet activation via Toll-like receptor 2. *J Thromb Haemost* 8:2757-2765.

Kerrigan, S.W., N. Clarke, A. Loughman, G. Meade, T.J. Foster, and D. Cox. 2008. Molecular basis for Staphylococcus aureus-mediated platelet aggregate formation under arterial shear in vitro. *Arterioscler Thromb Vasc Biol* 28:335-340.

Kerrigan, S.W., I. Douglas, A. Wray, J. Heath, M.F. Byrne, D. Fitzgerald, and D. Cox. 2002. A role for glycoprotein Ib in Streptococcus sanguis-induced platelet aggregation. *Blood* 100:509-516.

Kerrigan, S.W., N.S. Jakubovics, C. Keane, P. Maguire, K. Wynne, H.F. Jenkinson, and D. Cox. 2007. Role of Streptococcus gordonii surface proteins SspA/SspB and Hsa in platelet function. *Infect Immun* 75:5740-5747.

Lotz, S., A. Starke, C. Ziemann, S. Morath, T. Hartung, W. Solbach, and T. Laskay. 2006. Beta-lactam antibiotic-induced release of lipoteichoic acid from Staphylococcus aureus leads to activation of neutrophil granulocytes. *Ann Clin Microbiol Antimicrob* 5:15.

Loughman, A., J.R. Fitzgerald, M.P. Brennan, J. Higgins, R. Downer, D. Cox, and T.J. Foster. 2005. Roles for fibrinogen, immunoglobulin and complement in platelet activation promoted by Staphylococcus aureus clumping factor A. *Mol Microbiol* 57:804-818.

Lourbakos, A., Y.P. Yuan, A.L. Jenkins, J. Travis, P. Andrade-Gordon, R. Santulli, J. Potempa, and R.N. Pike. 2001. Activation of protease-activated receptors by gingipains from Porphyromonas gingivalis leads to platelet aggregation: a new trait in microbial pathogenicity. *Blood* 97:3790-3797.

Manohar, M., S.K. Maheswaran, S.P. Frommes, and R.K. Lindorfer. 1967. Platelet damaging factor, a fifth activity of staphylococcal alpha-toxin. *J Bacteriol* 94:224-231.

Marcus, A.J., H.L. Ullman, and L.B. Safier. 1972. Studies on human platelet gangliosides. *J Clin Invest* 51:2602-2612.

Matsumoto-Nakano, M., M. Tsuji, S. Inagaki, K. Fujita, K. Nagayama, R. Nomura, and T. Ooshima. 2009. Contribution of cell surface protein antigen c of Streptococcus mutans to platelet aggregation. *Oral Microbiol Immunol* 24:427-430.

McAleese, F.M., E.J. Walsh, M. Sieprawska, J. Potempa, and T.J. Foster. 2001. Loss of clumping factor B fibrinogen binding activity by Staphylococcus aureus involves cessation of transcription, shedding and cleavage by metalloprotease. *J Biol Chem* 276:29969-29978.

McNicol, A., R. Zhu, R. Pesun, C. Pampolina, E.C. Jackson, G.H. Bowden, and T. Zelinski. 2006. A role for immunoglobulin G in donor-specific Streptococcus sanguis-induced platelet aggregation. *Thromb Haemost* 95:288-293.

Meenan, N.A., L. Visai, V. Valtulina, U. Schwarz-Linek, N.C. Norris, S. Gurusiddappa, M. Hook, P. Speziale, and J.R. Potts. 2007. The tandem beta-zipper model defines high affinity fibronectin-binding repeats within Staphylococcus aureus FnBPA. *J Biol Chem* 282:25893-25902.

Mercier, R.-C., R.M. Dietz, J.L. Mazzola, A.S. Bayer, and M.R. Yeaman. 2004. Beneficial Influence of Platelets on Antibiotic Efficacy in an In Vitro Model of Staphylococcus aureus-Induced Endocarditis. *Antimicrob. Agents Chemother.* 48:2551-2557.

Miajlovic, H., A. Loughman, M. Brennan, D. Cox, and T.J. Foster. 2007. Both complement- and fibrinogen-dependent mechanisms contribute to platelet aggregation mediated by Staphylococcus aureus clumping factor B. *Infect Immun* 75:3335-3343.

Miajlovic, H., M. Zapotoczna, J.A. Geoghegan, S.W. Kerrigan, P. Speziale, and T.J. Foster. 2010. Direct interaction of iron-regulated surface determinant IsdB of Staphylococcus aureus with the GPIIb/IIIa receptor on platelets. *Microbiology* 156:920-928.

Mitchell, J., I.R. Siboo, D. Takamatsu, H.F. Chambers, and P.M. Sullam. 2007. Mechanism of cell surface expression of the Streptococcus mitis platelet binding proteins PblA and PblB. *Mol Microbiol* 64:844-857.

Morath, S., S. von Aulock, and T. Hartung. 2005. Structure/function relationships of lipoteichoic acids. *J Endotoxin Res* 11:348-356.

Moreillon, P., Y.A. Que, and A.S. Bayer. 2002. Pathogenesis of streptococcal and staphylococcal endocarditis. *Infect Dis Clin North Am* 16:297-318.

Moreillon, P.P., and Y.-A. Que. 2004. Infective endocarditis. *The Lancet* 363:139-149.

Motto, D.G., A.K. Chauhan, G. Zhu, J. Homeister, C.B. Lamb, K.C. Desch, W. Zhang, H.M. Tsai, D.D. Wagner, and D. Ginsburg. 2005. Shigatoxin triggers thrombotic thrombocytopenic purpura in genetically susceptible ADAMTS13-deficient mice. *J Clin Invest* 115:2752-2761.

Munro, C.L., and F.L. Macrina. 1993. Sucrose-derived exopolysaccharides of Streptococcus mutans V403 contribute to infectivity in endocarditis. *Mol Microbiol* 8:133-142.

Naber, C.K., and R. Erbel. 2007. Infective endocarditis with negative blood cultures. *International Journal of Antimicrobial Agents* 30:32-36.

Naito, M., E. Sakai, Y. Shi, H. Ideguchi, M. Shoji, N. Ohara, K. Yamamoto, and K. Nakayama. 2006. Porphyromonas gingivalis-induced platelet aggregation in plasma depends on Hgp44 adhesin but not Rgp proteinase. *Mol Microbiol* 59:152-167.

Nguyen, T., B. Ghebrehiwet, and E.I. Peerschke. 2000. Staphylococcus aureus protein A recognizes platelet gC1qR/p33: a novel mechanism for staphylococcal interactions with platelets. *Infect Immun* 68:2061-2068.

Nishimura, R.A., B.A. Carabello, D.P. Faxon, M.D. Freed, B.W. Lytle, P.T. O'Gara, R.A. O'Rourke, and P.M. Shah. 2008. ACC/AHA 2008 Guideline Update on Valvular Heart Disease: Focused Update on Infective Endocarditis. A Report of the American College of Cardiology/American Heart Association Task Force on Practice Guidelines. *Circulation* CIRCULATIONAHA.108.190377.

Nobbs, A.H., R.J. Lamont, and H.F. Jenkinson. 2009. Streptococcus adherence and colonization. *Microbiol Mol Biol Rev* 73:407-450, Table of Contents.

Nobbs, A.H., B.H. Shearer, M. Drobni, M.A. Jepson, and H.F. Jenkinson. 2007. Adherence and internalization of Streptococcus gordonii by epithelial cells involves beta1 integrin recognition by SspA and SspB (antigen I/II family) polypeptides. *Cell Microbiol* 9:65-83.

O'Seaghdha, M., C.J. van Schooten, S.W. Kerrigan, J. Emsley, G.J. Silverman, D. Cox, P.J. Lenting, and T.J. Foster. 2006. Staphylococcus aureus protein A binding to von Willebrand factor A1 domain is mediated by conserved IgG binding regions. *FEBS J* 273:4831-4841.

Ohkuni, H., Y. Todome, Y. Watanabe, S. Kotani, and Y. Kimura. 1997. Purification and partial characterization of a novel human platelet aggregation factor in the extracellular products of Streptococcus mitis, strain Nm-65. *Adv Exp Med Biol* 418:689-693.

Pampolina, C., and A. McNicol. 2005. Streptococcus sanguis-induced platelet activation involves two waves of tyrosine phosphorylation mediated by FcgammaRIIA and alphaIIbbeta3. *Thromb Haemost* 93:932-939.

Pawar, P., P.K. Shin, S.A. Mousa, J.M. Ross, and K. Konstantopoulos. 2004. Fluid shear regulates the kinetics and receptor specificity of Staphylococcus aureus binding to activated platelets. *J Immunol* 173:1258-1265.

Petersen, H.J., C. Keane, H.F. Jenkinson, M.M. Vickerman, A. Jesionowski, J.C. Waterhouse, D. Cox, and S.W. Kerrigan. 2010. Human platelets recognize a novel surface protein, PadA, on Streptococcus gordonii through a unique interaction involving fibrinogen receptor GPIIbIIIa. *Infect Immun* 78:413-422.

Plummer, C., H. Wu, S.W. Kerrigan, G. Meade, D. Cox, and C.W. Ian Douglas. 2005. A serine-rich glycoprotein of Streptococcus sanguis mediates adhesion to platelets via GPIb. *Br J Haematol* 129:101-109.

Prakobphol, A., F. Xu, V.M. Hoang, T. Larsson, J. Bergstrom, I. Johansson, L. Frangsmyr, U. Holmskov, H. Leffler, C. Nilsson, T. Boren, J.R. Wright, N. Stromberg, and S.J. Fisher. 2000. Salivary agglutinin, which binds Streptococcus mutans and Helicobacter pylori, is the lung scavenger receptor cysteine-rich protein gp-340. *J Biol Chem* 275:39860-39866.

Raibaud, S., U. Schwarz-Linek, J.H. Kim, H.T. Jenkins, E.R. Baines, S. Gurusiddappa, M. Hook, and J.R. Potts. 2005. Borrelia burgdorferi binds fibronectin through a tandem beta-zipper, a common mechanism of fibronectin binding in staphylococci, streptococci, and spirochetes. *J Biol Chem* 280:18803-18809.

Ramboarina, S., J.A. Garnett, M. Zhou, Y. Li, Z. Peng, J.D. Taylor, W.C. Lee, A. Bodey, J.W. Murray, Y. Alguel, J. Bergeron, B. Bardiaux, E. Sawyer, R. Isaacson, C. Tagliaferri, E. Cota, M. Nilges, P. Simpson, T. Ruiz, H. Wu, and S. Matthews. 2010. Structural insights into serine-rich fimbriae from Gram-positive bacteria. *J Biol Chem* 285:32446-32457.

Rasmussen, M., D. Johansson, S.K. Sobirk, M. Morgelin, and O. Shannon. 2010. Clinical isolates of Enterococcus faecalis aggregate human platelets. *Microbes Infect* 12:295-301.

Rasmussen, R.V., U. Host, M. Arpi, C. Hassager, H.K. Johansen, E. Korup, H.C. Schonheyder, J. Berning, S. Gill, F.S. Rosenvinge, V.G. Fowler, Jr., J.E. Moller, R.L. Skov, C.T. Larsen, T.F. Hansen, S. Mard, J. Smit, P.S. Andersen, and N.E. Bruun. 2011. Prevalence of infective endocarditis in patients with Staphylococcus aureus bacteraemia: the value of screening with echocardiography. *Eur J Echocardiogr* 12:414-420.

Ruggeri, Z.M. 2009. Platelet adhesion under flow. *Microcirculation* 16:58-83.

Schwarz, S., A. Bottner, H.M. Hafez, C. Kehrenberg, M. Kietzmann, D. Klarmann, G. Klein, P. Krabisch, T. Kuhn, G. Luhofer, A. Richter, W. Traeder, K.H. Waldmann, J. Wallmann, and C. Werckenthin. 2003. [Antimicrobial susceptibility testing of bacteria isolated from animals: methods for in-vitro susceptibility testing and their suitability with regard to the generation of the most useful data for therapeutic applications]. *Berl Munch Tierarztl Wochenschr* 116:353-361.

Semple, J., and J. Freedman. 2010. Platelets and innate immunity. *Cellular and Molecular Life Sciences* 67:499-511.

Seo, H.S., Y.Q. Xiong, J. Mitchell, R. Seepersaud, A.S. Bayer, and P.M. Sullam. 2010. Bacteriophage lysin mediates the binding of streptococcus mitis to human platelets through interaction with fibrinogen. *PLoS Pathog* 6:

Sheu, J.R., G. Hsiao, C. Lee, W. Chang, L.W. Lee, C.H. Su, and C.H. Lin. 2000a. Antiplatelet activity of Staphylococcus aureus lipoteichoic acid is mediated through a cyclic AMP pathway. *Thromb Res* 99:249-258.

Sheu, J.R., C.R. Lee, C.H. Lin, G. Hsiao, W.C. Ko, Y.C. Chen, and M.H. Yen. 2000b. Mechanisms involved in the antiplatelet activity of Staphylococcus aureus lipoteichoic acid in human platelets. *Thromb Haemost* 83:777-784.

Siboo, I.R., H.F. Chambers, and P.M. Sullam. 2005. Role of SraP, a Serine-Rich Surface
    Protein of Staphylococcus aureus, in binding to human platelets. *Infect Immun*
    73:2273-2280.
Siegel, I., and S. Cohen. 1964. Action of Staphylococcal Toxin on Human Platelets. *J Infect Dis*
    114:488-502.
Skaar, E.P., and O. Schneewind. 2004. Iron-regulated surface determinants (Isd) of
    Staphylococcus aureus: stealing iron from heme. *Microbes Infect* 6:390-397.
Sullam, P.M., A.S. Bayer, W.M. Foss, and A.L. Cheung. 1996. Diminished platelet binding in
    vitro by Staphylococcus aureus is associated with reduced virulence in a rabbit
    model of infective endocarditis. *Infect Immun* 64:4915-4921.
Takahashi, Y., K. Konishi, J.O. Cisar, and M. Yoshikawa. 2002. Identification and
    characterization of hsa, the gene encoding the sialic acid-binding adhesin of
    Streptococcus gordonii DL1. *Infect Immun* 70:1209-1218.
Takahashi, Y., A. Yajima, J.O. Cisar, and K. Konishi. 2004. Functional analysis of the
    Streptococcus gordonii DL1 sialic acid-binding adhesin and its essential role in
    bacterial binding to platelets. *Infect Immun* 72:3876-3882.
Takamatsu, D., B.A. Bensing, H. Cheng, G.A. Jarvis, I.R. Siboo, J.A. Lopez, J.M. Griffiss, and
    P.M. Sullam. 2005. Binding of the Streptococcus gordonii surface glycoproteins
    GspB and Hsa to specific carbohydrate structures on platelet membrane
    glycoprotein Ibalpha. *Mol Microbiol* 58:380-392.
Valeva, A., A. Weisser, B. Walker, M. Kehoe, H. Bayley, S. Bhakdi, and M. Palmer. 1996.
    Molecular architecture of a toxin pore: a 15-residue sequence lines the
    transmembrane channel of staphylococcal alpha-toxin. *EMBO J* 15:1857-1864.
Vanhoorelbeke, K., H. Ulrichts, G. Van de Walle, A. Fontayne, and H. Deckmyn. 2007.
    Inhibition of platelet glycoprotein Ib and its antithrombotic potential. *Curr Pharm
    Des* 13:2684-2697.
Varki, A. 1994. Selectin ligands. *Proc Natl Acad Sci U S A* 91:7390-7397.
Viisoreanu, D., R. Polanowska-Grabowska, S. Suttitanamongkol, T.G. Obrig, and A.R. Gear.
    2000. Human platelet aggregation is not altered by Shiga toxins 1 or 2. *Thromb Res*
    98:403-410.
Ward, J.R., L. Bingle, H.M. Judge, S.B. Brown, R.F. Storey, M.K. Whyte, S.K. Dower, D.J.
    Buttle, and I. Sabroe. 2005. Agonists of toll-like receptor (TLR)2 and TLR4 are
    unable to modulate platelet activation by adenosine diphosphate and platelet
    activating factor. *Thromb Haemost* 94:831-838.
Wu, H., M. Zeng, and P. Fives-Taylor. 2007. The glycan moieties and the N terminal
    polypeptide backbone of a fimbria-associated adhesin, Fap1, play distinct roles in
    the biofilm development of Streptococcus parasanguinis. *Infect Immun* 75:2181-
    2188.
Yajima, A., Y. Takahashi, and K. Konishi. 2005. Identification of platelet receptors for the
    Streptococcus gordonii DL1 sialic acid-binding adhesin. *Microbiol Immunol* 49:795-
    800.
Youssefian, T., A. Drouin, J.M. Masse, J. Guichard, and E.M. Cramer. 2002. Host defense role
    of platelets: engulfment of HIV and Staphylococcus aureus occurs in a specific
    subcellular compartment and is enhanced by platelet activation. *Blood* 99:4021-4029.
Zahringer, U., B. Lindner, S. Inamura, H. Heine, and C. Alexander. 2008. TLR2 -
    promiscuous or specific? A critical re-evaluation of a receptor expressing apparent
    broad specificity. *Immunobiology* 213:205-224.

4

Infective Endocarditis in the Elderly

Lucy Miller and Jim George
Department of Medicine for the Elderly,
Cumberland Infirmary, Carlisle,
U.K.

1. Introduction

In the 21st century, despite advanced diagnostic imaging, improved antibiotic treatment, and widely available surgery, the incidence of infective endocarditis (IE) has not reduced in recent years, and continues to have high morbidity and mortality (Prendergast, 2005). Over the years there have been changes in the natural history, predisposing factors, sequelae and causative organisms. In particular, rheumatic heart disease is an uncommon predisposing factor, and now degenerative valve disease is much more common in the elderly population. As with many conditions, elderly patients with IE can present in very non-specific ways, making diagnosis more difficult, leading to delays in treatment. IE in elderly patients is associated with a poor prognosis. Fewer patients receive valve surgery, due to higher operative risk, but this does still remain a treatment option for suitable patients. Our knowledge and understanding of endocarditis in the elderly, compared to younger patients, is predominantly influenced by important case series reports in the literature (Table 1) and these will be referred to in the text. European Guidelines are available for guidance in management of IE in all age groups (European Society of Cardiology, 2009).

2. Epidemiology

Elderly patients are predisposed to infectious diseases for multiple reasons; impairment of innate and adaptive immunity, increased comorbidities, increased functional limitations, increased instrumentation and implantation of prosthetic devices, and increased numbers of patients living in care homes (High et al, 2005). These factors result in an increase in adverse outcomes in the elderly. It therefore stands to reason that the incidence of IE has been shown to increase with age, and the incidence amongst elderly patients is also increasing (Dhawan, 2002). So with the ageing population, IE in the elderly is at an all time high. In the European Heart Survey, 26% of cases of IE were in elderly patients (>70 years old) (Iung et al, 2003), and in a French survey 33% of IE patients were over 67 years of age (Delahaye et al, 1999). In further French studies, the incidence of IE peaked between the ages of 70 and 80 years (Hoen et al, 2002). The risk of IE in the elderly has been found to be 4.6 times higher than in the general population. Reasons for this may include a high prevalence of undiagnosed degenerative valve disease, and again higher rates of invasive procedures and implanted devices compared to younger patients.

Author	Patients		Clinical features	Prosthetic devices (e.g. pacemakers or valves)	Causes	Surgery	Mortality
Selton-Suty et al (1997)	Total Over 70 Under 70	114 25 89	Younger patients more embolic complications 28% v 8% (p< 0.05)	52% elderly v 25% young (p< 0.05)	Portal of entry more often digestive in older patients 50% v 17% (p=0.01)	Older patients less often operated on 24% v 43% (p=0.07)	Mortality higher in older patients 28% v 13% (p=0.08)
Di Salvo et al (2003)	Total Over 70 50-70 Under 50	315 87 111 117	Clinical features similar between 3 groups except anaemia less common in patients under 50 years	Pacemaker endocarditis commoner in over 70's, but prosthetic valve endocarditis similar in both groups	Older patients more often digestive or urinary portal of entry	50% under 50 years, 52% 50-70, 41% over 70 (p=0.35)	10% under 50 years, 7% 50-70, 17% over 70 (p=0.02)
Durante-Mangoni et al (2008)	Total Over 65 Under 65	2759 1056 1703	Mitral valve involvement more common in older people. Fewer vegetations and more abscesses in older patients. Vascular and immune mediated phenomena, including embolisation, less common in older people (p<0.001). Chronic illnesses, including diabetes and cancer, commoner in older people. Rate of complications lower in older people.	More commonly prosthetic devices or pacemakers in older people (p<0.001)	MRSA, Strep bovis and enterococci more common in older patients	38.5% older v 53.5% younger (p<0.001)	24.9% older v 12.8% younger. Age an independent predictor of mortality.
Remadi et al (2009)	Total Over 75 Under 75	348 75 273	Older patients more severely ill and more comorbidities. No difference in embolism risk.	Pacemakers and prosthetic valve endocarditis significantly more common in older patients (p<0.001)	Similar between older and younger patients	29% older v 56% younger (p=0.001)	No significant difference between young and old
Ramirez-Duque et al (2011)	Total Over 65 Under 65	961 356 605	Comorbidity, renal failure and septic shock more common in older patients	25% older patients v 23% young patients (NS)	Nosocomial acquisition commoner in older patients (p<0.01)	36% older v 51% younger (p<0.01)	42% older v 26% younger (p0.01)

Table 1. Case series of infective endocarditis in older people compared to the young

It has been previously reported that IE in the elderly is associated with a poor prognosis and high complication rate. The onset is usually insidious, sometimes the presenting symptoms are less severe, and diagnosis is sometimes therefore delayed, as well as more aggressive pathogens causing the infection. Age has been shown to be an independent prognostic factor for in-hospital mortality (Durante-Mangoni et al, 2008).

3. Causes

Historically, previous rheumatic heart disease was a very common predisposing factor for IE (Prendergast, 2005). However, this is now rarely a factor. Older people are particularly prone to develop mitral annular calcium (MAC). This is a chronic degenerative process that occurs in older persons, particularly women, and often results in mitral regurgitation (Roberts and Perloff, 1972). Older people with MAC have a high incidence of atrial fibrillation and are especially at risk of developing endocarditis (Mambo et al, 1978). The avascular nature of the mitral annulus prevents antibiotics reaching the bacteria, predisposing to peri annular abscesses and a poor prognosis. Aronow et al (1990) demonstrated at follow up of 39 months a 3% incidence of bacterial endocarditis in 526 older persons with MAC and only a 1% incidence in 450 older persons without MAC. In IE in the elderly, gastrointestinal sources of bacteria are more common. Group D streptococcus (Streptococcus bovis) is frequently implicated (Vahanian, 2003). This is associated with colonic pathology, in particular neoplasia, as well as the involvement of multiple valves and embolic complications. Enterococcus is also more common in the elderly. However, it has also been reported that vegetations in the elderly are generally smaller, with a lower embolic risk (Selton-Suty et al, 1997). Pathogens are more commonly of urinary origin as well. It is thought that this is due to the higher proportion of urethral and prostatic procedures performed in the elderly (Di Salvo et al, 2003). Pacemaker endocarditis is commoner amongst the elderly, as would be expected as the number of patients with pacemakers increases with age (Remadi et al, 2009). Pacemaker endocarditis has been associated with even more difficult and delayed diagnosis, resulting in a poor prognosis.

4. Diagnosis

The clinical diagnosis of IE is based on Duke criteria, which includes positive blood cultures, suggestive features on echocardiography, predisposing heart disease, fever, and vascular and immunological phenomena (Prendergast, 2005). The St Thomas modifications include serology, elevated inflammatory markers, and other clinical signs including splenomegaly, haematuria, splinter haemorrhages and rashes (Prendergast, 2005). However, the onset of IE can be acute or insidious, and the presence of classical signs as described by Duke criteria are often absent, particularly in the elderly (Vahanian, 2003). Therefore, in the presence of signs of sepsis with no obvious source, IE should always be considered in the elderly. Table 2 lists the many common presentations in older people. Overall, the elderly report fewer symptoms (Selton-Suty, 1997). Fever is less common than with younger patients, but anaemia is more common, probably due to the presence of Streptococcus bovis and colonic pathology, resulting in bleeding and anaemia. Delirium is also a more prominent feature. Murmurs are often thought to be insignificant in the elderly, so do not necessarily raise suspicion of IE. New or changing murmurs are heard less frequently in the elderly. Positive blood cultures remain the main diagnostic tool (Prendergast, 2005). At least three sets of cultures should be taken prior to the administration of any antibiotics, and ideally both aerobic and anaerobic cultures should be incubated. Negative cultures most frequently occur after prior antibiotic administration, but increasingly due to fastidious organisms. In particular, negative cultures occur in IE related to prosthetic valves and pacemakers, which are more common in the elderly. Transthoracic and transoesophageal echocardiography (TTE and TOE respectively) are now commonly used in the diagnosis and management of IE (Prendergast, 2005). It has been reported that the detection of vegetations in the elderly is lower with TTE, so TOE should be used as it is more sensitive and specific. In general, TTE is performed first, then TOE performed when TTE is negative, but there is a high clinical suspicion of IE. TOE has revolutionised the diagnosis of IE in the elderly by increasing the diagnostic yield by 45% (Dhawan, 2002).

Sepsis of unknown origin (especially if associated with known infective endocarditis causative organism). New regurgitant murmur. Embolic events of unknown origin. Fever if associated with:

- Intracardiac prosthetic material, including pacemakers

- Previous valvular heart disease

- Congestive cardiac failure

- Recent medical interventions with bacteraemia New cardiac conduction disturbance

- Positive blood cultures with IE causative organism

- Peripheral abscesses of unknown cause

- Non specific neurological symptoms or signs

- Previous history of IE

Table 2. Clinical presentations of infective endocarditis in the elderly

5. Management

Successful treatment of IE in the elderly requires close cooperation between the geriatrician, cardiologist, microbiologist, and cardiac surgeon. Regular review of the patient is required to assess for progression or development of complications (Prendergast, 2005). International guidelines have been published to provide recommendations on the treatment of IE (European Society of Cardiology, 2009). Rapid administration of antibiotics is critical in the initial management of IE (Dhawan, 2002). Antibiotics in high serum concentrations are essential to ensure penetration into the vegetations, and prolonged treatment (4-6 weeks) is required to kill dormant bacteria (Prendergast, 2005). Intravenous antibiotics as an in-patient is the preferred method, but with increasing provision for the administration of intravenous antibiotics in the community, this is becoming an increasingly popular option after the initial two week treatment period when the complication rate is highest. However, this may not be a suitable option in elderly patients who may require in-patient care for the full duration of treatment. Usual initial treatment is broad spectrum, with a combination of a penicillin and an aminoglycoside. In the presence of a prosthetic valve vancomycin or gentamicin is usually used, with or without rifampicin (Dhawan, 2002). There is no evidence for the use of oral antibiotics after the completion of the intravenous course (Prendergast, 2005). When IE is suspected, and after blood cultures have been taken, broad spectrum intravenous antibiotics should be administered until the results of the cultures and sensitivities is known, then a more specific antibiotic can be commenced (Prendergast, 2005). Prosthetic valve and pacemaker endocarditis, which is more common in the elderly requires 4-6 weeks of intravenous antibiotics, as well as removal of the prosthesis if possible (Prendergast, 2005). Repeat valve surgery is recommended in early prosthetic valve endocarditis. Surgery can be life saving in cases of IE and has been shown to be of benefit in suitable elderly patients. Often elderly patients are more unwell with multiple comorbidities and therefore may be deemed unsuitable for surgery (Prendergast, 2005). In one study (Di Salvo et al, 2003) surgery was performed only slightly less frequently than in younger patients and the operated group had a lower mortality. Of course this may reflect the fact that the patients suitable for surgery are generally fitter. Elderly patients may also refuse surgery. In a recent study of 961 patients with endocarditis in Spain (Ramírez-Duque, 2011) significantly fewer elderly patients underwent cardiac surgery (Table 1). The three main indications for surgery are heart failure, uncontrolled infection, and prevention of embolic events (European Society of Cardiology, 2009). In the Spanish study (Ramírez-Duque, 2011), compared with medical treatment, surgery showed lower mortality in the younger patients (less than 65 years), but a high mortality was observed with both medical and surgical treatment in the elderly (over 65 years). Overall in Europe, surgery is undertaken in around 50% of patients with IE with long-term survival rates of around 70% (Prendergast and Tornos, 2010). Surgery is better undertaken early before cardiac tissue damage has occurred and there is a general deterioration in the patients condition. Delay in surgery may contribute to poor outcomes in older patients.

6. Culture negative endocarditis in the elderly

Culture negative endocarditis is particularly common in older patients. The definition of culture negative endocarditis is endocarditis which fulfils established diagnostic criteria for endocarditis, but at least three independent blood cultures are negative after seven days of incubation and subculturing (Raoult et al, 2005). A two year multicentre prospective study in Italy found that 25% of patients with a definite diagnosis of endocarditis by Duke criteria were culture-negative (Cecchi et al, 2004). Cultures are negative in endocarditis for three major reasons: i) previous administration of antibiotics; ii) inadequate microbiological techniques, or iii) infection with highly fastidious bacteria or non-bacterial pathogens (e.g. fungi). Risk factors for culture negative endocarditis include underlying valvular heart disease, presence of a pacemaker and exposure to fastidious organisms. HACEK organisms (Haemophilus aphrophilus; Actinobacillus actinomycetemcomitans; Cardiobacterium hominis; Eikenella corrodens and Kingella Kingae) were originally thought to be the most common cause. However, better laboratory techniques have now led to the more successful isolation of these organisms. In a prospective study of 348 patients with culture negative endocarditis 275 (79%) aetiological agents were identified using serological tests, and polymerase chain reaction (PCR) techniques (Houpikian and Raoult, 2005). The commonest agents found were coxiella burnetti (Q fever) and bartonella species. Serology and PCR on blood samples or removed valves can therefore help considerably in identifying fastidious organisms. Fungi are particularly common pathogens in early prosthetic valve endocarditis (Thuny et al, 2010). Clinically if it is not possible to identify the aetiological agent then treatment may have to be directed either at the most likely source if the patient has already been on antibiotics, or as broad spectrum as possible while closely monitoring clinical response. The long-term prognosis of negative blood culture IE in the elderly is similar to patients with positive blood cultures (Peréz de Isla et al, 2007). A specific form of culture negative endocarditis can occur in older people and cause diagnostic uncertainty. Non-bacterial thrombotic endocarditis (NBTE), or marantic endocarditis, is a rare condition associated with cancer and other illnesses where there is an increased thrombotic tendency, for example septicaemia (Clough et al, 2010). Clinical features of NBTE are very small, multiple valvular vegetations which may be only visible on TOE and multiple small, medium and large disseminated emboli in patients with an underlying cause for NBTE , and multiple negative blood cultures and serology. NBTE, unlike IE, may benefit from anticoagulation, but the outlook is poor, usually because of the underlying cause.

7. Complications and outcomes of infective endocarditis in the elderly

Complications of infective endocarditis can be categorised as:

i.   cardiac;
ii. septic;
iii. embolic;
iv. neurological;
v.   musculoskeletal;
vi. renal;
vii. associated with medical treatment.

Cardiac complications are the most common complication in older patients. The most common of these is heart failure which is also the most common cause of death in IE. The usual cause of heart failure is infection-induced valvular damage for which cardiac surgery may be lifesaving. Embolisation seems less common in older people (Selton-Suty, 1997), but can occur resulting in stroke, splenic or renal infarction or myocardial infarction. The risk of embolisation is reduced by prompt antibiotic therapy. Apart from embolic stroke, other neurological complications include brain abscesses, seizures, meningitis and encephalitis. Renal failure may result from renal infarction, but also from glomerulonephritis and rarely renal abscesses. Musculoskeletal complications include vertebral osteomyelitis or discitis and septic arthritis. Finally, older patients with IE can develop complications associated with prolonged antibiotic treatment – for example ototoxicity and nephrotoxicity. It is widely accepted that age is an independent predictor of mortality in IE (Durante-Mangoni et al, 2008). Other factors associated with poor outcome are listed in Table 3 and include diabetes, significant comorbidities, heart failure and echocardiographic findings of poor left ventricular function, severe valve regurgitation and large vegetations. However, prognostic predictions should be made with caution in individual patients and many of these factors may be correctable with surgery.

8. Prevention of endocarditis in the elderly

It has previously been recommended that antibiotic prophylaxis should be given to the majority of patients with congenital and valvular heart disease before any dental or surgical procedure. However, this recommendation has now been narrowed to only high risk patients, including patients with prosthetic heart valves or with a previous history of IE and only for high risk procedures. High risk procedures include dental procedures that involve manipulation of gingival tissue, or the peri-apical region of the teeth, or perforation of the oral mucosa and also procedures in patients with ongoing gastrointestinal or genito-urinary infections. Interestingly, the NICE guidelines for England and Wales do not advocate antibiotics, even for high risk patients undergoing dental procedures (Chambers et al, 2011). This is because of lack of convincing trial evidence for antibiotic prophylaxis, even in this high risk group, and the risk of anaphylaxis with antibiotics and the potential development of antibiotic resistance. However, this is contrary to the European guidelines (European Society of Cardiology, 2009) and the usual practice of most clinicians who are influenced by the high mortality rate of high risk patients if they develop endocarditis, even though it may be a rare complication.

Older age Prosthetic valve endocarditis Diabetes Comorbidity (frailty, renal or pulmonary disease) Complications
- heart failure
- renal failure
- stroke
- septic shock Infecting organisms
- staphylococcus aureus
- fungi
- gram negative bacilli Echocardiographic findings
- large vegetations
- pulmonary hypertension
- periannular complications
- poor left ventricular ejection fraction
- severe left sided valve regurgitation or severe prosthetic dysfunction

Table 3. Predictors of poor outcome in older patients with infective endocarditis

9. Conclusion

IE is a very important and atypical illness in older people. Firstly, its incidence seems to be increasing because of the increase in degenerative valvular disease and the increasing use of cardiac prosthetic devices. Secondly, it can present in a variety of different ways depending on the underlying cardiac disease and the microorganisms involved and the underlying patient comorbidities and resistance to infection. It therefore requires a collaborative approach involving physicians, geriatricians, cardiologists, cardiac surgeons and microbiologists. Thirdly, the evidence for its clinical manifestations, treatment and prognosis comes from clinical case series rather than from clinical trials or meta-analyses. Five important case series predominantly from Europe have been published and are summarised in Table 1, comparing older patients with younger patients with IE. Consistently older patients tend to have a higher mortality, are less likely to have surgery and more likely to have prosthetic devices and be infected with bacteria from the gut or urinary tract. Older people are more likely to present insidiously with smaller vegetations and less embolic manifestations. It can be argued that IE is a completely different disease in the older person and deserves a different, more aggressive approach in both treatment and prevention because of its high morbidity and mortality.

10. References

Aronow, W.S., Koenigsberg, M., Kronzon, I. et al (1990). "Association of mitral annular calcification with new thromboembolic stroke and cardiac events at 39-month follow up in elderly patients." *Am J Cardiol*; 65: 1511-1512. Cecchi, E., Forno, D., Imazio, M., Migliardi,

A., Gnavi, R., Dal Conte, I. & Trinchero, R. (2004). "New trends in the epidemiological and clinical features of infective endocarditis: results of a multicenter prospective study." *Ital Heart ;J* Apr;5(4): 249-56.

Chambers, J.B., Shanson, D., Hall, R., Pepper, J., Graham V. & McGurk, M. (2011). "Antibiotic prophylaxis of endocarditis: the rest of the world and NICE." *J R Soc Med*; 104: 138-140.

Clough, H., George, J. & Duncan, A. (2010). "Psychosis due to non-bacterial thrombotic endocarditis." *Age and Ageing*; 39: 276-277.

Delahye, F., Rial, M.O., de Gevigney, G., Ecochard, R. & Delaye, J. (1999). "A critical appraisal of the quality of the management of infective endocarditis." *J Am Coll Cardiol*; 33: 788-793.

Di Salvo, G., Thuny, F., Rosenberg, V., Pergola, V., Belliard, O., Derumeaux, G., Cohen, A., Larussi, D., Giorgi, R., Casalta, J.P., Caso, P. & Habib, G. (2003). "Endocarditis in the elderly: clinical echocardiographic, and prognostic features." *European Heart Journal*; 24: 1576-1583.

Dhawan, V.K. (2002). "Infective Endocarditis in Elderly Patients." *Clinical Infectious Diseases*; 34 (15 March): 806-812.

Durante-Mangoni, E., Bradley, S., Selton-Suty, C., Gripodi, M.F., Barsic, B., Bouza, E., Cabell, C.H., de Oliveira Ramos, A.I., Fowler, V., Hoen, B., Konecny, P., Morena, A., Murdoch, D., Pappas, P., Sexton, D.J., Spelman, D., Tattevin, P., Miró, J.M., van der Meer, J.T.M. & Utili, R. (2008). "Current Features of Infective Endocarditis in Elderly Patients." *Arch Intern Med*; 168(19): 2095-2103.

European Society of Cardiology' (2009). "Guidelines on the prevention, diagnosis, and treatment of infective endocarditis (new version 2009)." *European Heart Journal*; 30: 2369-2413.

High, K.P., Bradley, S., Loeb, M., Palmer, R., Quagiarello, V. & Yoshikawa, T. (2005). "A New Paradigm for Clinical Investigation of Infectious Syndromes in Older Adults: Assessment of Functional Status as a Risk Factor and Outcome Measure." *Clinical Infectious Diseases*; 40: 114-122.

Hoen, B., Alla, F., Selton-Suty, C., Beguinot, I., Bouvet, A., Briancon, S., Casalta, J.P., Danchin, N., Delahaye, F., Etienne, J., LeMoing, V., Leport, C., Mainard, J.C., Rulmy, R. & Vandenesch, F. (2002). "Changing profile of infective endocarditis: results of a 1-year survey in France." *JAMA*; 288: 75-81.

Houpikian, P. & Raoult, D. (2005). "Blood culture-negative endocarditis in a reference center: etiologic diagnosis of 348 cases." *Medicine (Baltimore)*, May; 84(3): 162-173.

Iung, B., Baron, G., Butchart, E.G., Delahaye, F., Gohlke-Barwolf, C., Levang, O.W., Tornos, P., Vanoverschelde, J.L., Vermeer, F., Boersma, E., Ravaud, P. & Vahanian, A. (2003). "A prospective survey of patients with valvular heart disease in Europe: the Euro Heart Survey on Valvular Heart Disease. *Eur Heart J*; 24: 1231- 1243.

Mambo, W.C., Silver, M.D., Brunsdon, D.F.V. (1978). "Bacterial endocarditis of the mitral valve associated with annular calcification." *Can Med Assoc J*; 119: 323-326.

Peréz de Isla, L., Zamorano, J., Lennie, V., Vázquez, J., Ribera, J.M. & Macaya, C. (2007). "Negative Blood Culture Infective Endocarditis in the Elderly: Long-Term Follow Up." *Gerontology*; 53: 245-249.

Prendergast, B.D. (2006). "The changing face of infective endocarditis.". *Heart*; 92: 879-885.

Prendergast, B.D. & Tornos, P. (2010). "Surgery for Infective Endocarditis: Who and When?" *Circulation*; 121: 1141-1152.

Ramírez-Duque, E., Carcía-Cabrera, R., Ivanova-Georgieva, R., Noureddine, M., Lomas, J.M., Hidalgo-Tenorio, A., Plata, J., Gálvez-Acebal, J., Ruíz-Morales, J., de la Torre-Lima, J., Reguera, J.M., Martínez-Marcos, F.J. & de Alarcón, A. (2011). "Surgical treatment for infective endocarditis in elderly patients." *Journal of Infection*; 63: 131-138.

Raoult, D., Casalta, J.P., Richet, H., Khan, M., Bernit, E., Rovery, C., Branger, S., Gouriet, F., Imbert, G., Bothello, E., Cocllart, F. & Habib, G. (2005). "Contribution of systematic serological testing in diagnosis of infective endocarditis." *J Clin Microbiol.*, Oct:43(10): 5238-5242.

Remadi, J.P., Nadji, G., Goissen, T., Zomvuama, N.A., Sorel, C. & Tribouilloy, C. (2009). "Infective endocarditis in elderly patients: clinical characteristics and outcome." *Eur J Cardiothorac Surg*; 35: 123-129.

Roberts, W.C., Perloff, J.K. (1972). "Mitral valvular disease. A clinicopathologic survey of the conditions causing the mitral valve to function normally." *Ann Intern Med*; 77: 939-975.

Selton-Suty, C., Hoen, B., Grentzinger, A., Houplon, P., Maignan, M., Juilliére, Y., Danchin, N., Canton, P. & Cherrier, F. (1997). "Clinical and bacteriological characteristics of infective endocarditis in the elderly." *Heart*; 77: 260-263.

Thuny, F., Fournier, P.E., Casalta, J.P., Gouriet, F., Lepidi, H., Riberi, A., Collart, F., Habib, G. & Raoult, D. (2010). "Investigation of blood culture-negative early prosthetic valve endocarditis reveals high prevalence of fungi." *Heart,* May;96(10): 743-747.

Vahanian, A. (2003). "The growing burden of infective endocarditis in the elderly." *European Heart Journal;* 24: 1539-1540.

5

Antibiotics Against Endocarditis – Past, Present and Future (Experimental Data)

Cédric Jacqueline, Gilles Amador, Eric Batard,
Virginie Le Mabecque, Gilles Potel and Jocelyne Caillon
Université de Nantes, Faculté de Médecine, UPRES EA 3826, Nantes
France

1. Introduction

"Bacterial infections are becoming increasingly resistant to existing antibiotics, and as the number of patients who have succumbed to these infections rises, the number of new antibiotics being developed continues to plummet." This extract from a letter addressed to President Barack Obama by the president of Infectious Diseases Society of America (IDSA) attests to the urgent need for new therapeutic options to fight multidrug-resistant (MDR) bacteria. Drug-resistant infections and related morbidity and mortality are on the rise in the United States and around the world. Despite the growing antibiotic resistance among Gram-positive and Gram-negative pathogens causing severe infections in hospital and community settings, the number of new antibacterial drugs approved for marketing in the United States continues to decrease. In addition to this worrying situation, only a few novel therapeutics for drug-resistant infections are in the drug development pipeline (Boucher et al., 2009; European Centre for Disease Prevention and Control, 2009). Reports of bacterial isolates resistant to almost all available antibiotics highlight the crucial need for new antibiotic therapies, especially for Gram-negative infections (Maltezou, 2009). Recently, IDSA and United States authorities have developed creative incentives to stimulate new antibacterial research and development (Infectious Diseases Society of America, 2010).

In vivo assessment is recognized as an essential link between in vitro data such as susceptibility testing and clinical studies. As indicated in 1999 in the introduction to the Handbook of Animal Models of Infection (Zak et al., 1999), it is hardly conceivable that a new antibiotic could move into clinical use without thorough verification of its antimicrobial efficacy in animal models of infection at an early stage. To facilitate the extrapolation of animal model data to humans, especially for determination of efficacy, animal models mimicking human disease are required. Pharmacokinetic (PK) and pharmacodynamic (PD) features of new antibacterial agents must be considered and differences between PK of antibiotics in animals and human should be limited using methods for obtaining human-like PK profiles in animals. Animal models mimicking human infections are considered discriminative models and are designed to assess the potent therapeutic effects of antibiotics against pathogens, and in some cases to extend or delimit the indications advisable for humans.

Animal models of endocarditis are used extensively to test the in vivo activities of new drugs or new regimens, and are particularly suitable for PK and PD analysis and optimization of therapeutic efficacy. Experimental endocarditis studies played a major role in the exploration and assessment of new antistaphylococcal drugs beginning with the oxazolidinone, linezolid, in the early 2000s, and were critical to the recent approval of the promising anti-MRSA cephalosporin ceftaroline by the United States Food and Drug Administration (FDA). The endocarditis model is referenced in approximately 100 PubMed publications, most of which are assessments of the in vivo activity of new therapeutic options against *Staphylococcus aureus* such as linezolid (Jacqueline et al., 2002), quinupristin-dalfopristin (Batard et al., 2002), moxifloxacin (Entenza et al., 2001), daptomycin (Sakoulas et al., 2003), tigecycline (Murphy et al., 2000; Jacqueline et al., 2011), ceftobiprole (Tattevin et al., 2010) and ceftaroline (Jacqueline et al., 2007). *Staphylococcus aureus* is the most common cause of endocarditis worldwide and methicillin-susceptible *Staphylococcus aureus* (MSSA) is detected in up to two-thirds of cases (Fowler et al., 2005). High rates of clinical failure have been reported with vancomycin therapy for MRSA endocarditis. The emergence of glycopeptide-intermediate *Staphylococcus aureus* (GISA) strains further highlights the need for new therapeutic options for treatment of infections by *S. aureus* strains that are resistant to methicillin and glycopeptides.

Ideally, clinicians should be able to use clinical trial data to support evidence-based medicine for the treatment of infectious diseases. However, difficulty in performing clinical trials in severe types of infection such as endocarditis has resulted in a lack of clinical information regarding use of new antibiotics in treating severe infections. Experimental animal models are one method used to assess the in vivo activity of new antimicrobials in the treatment of severe infections.

2. Experimental model of endocarditis: How to?

Although experimental rodent endocarditis models are sometimes used, white New Zealand female (weighing 2-2.5 kg) are most commonly used in experimental studies involving evaluation of antimicrobial agents. This model is based on the description by Garrison and Freedman in 1970 (Garrison & Freedman, 1970) modified by Durack and Beeson in 1972 (Durack & Beeson, 1972).

The rabbit model, as currently used, is based on the insertion of a polyethylene catheter via the right carotid artery into the left ventricle under general anaesthesia. The catheter is left in place throughout the experiment (until the euthanasia of the animal). After catherization for 24 hours, each animal is inoculated i.v. (using the marginal ear vein) with 1 mL of a bacterial suspension of the test pathogen. The inoculum is usually prepared from an overnight culture (broth), centrifuged and calibrated in saline to the appropriate dilution (range, 10^5 to 10^9 CFU/mL). Bacterial concentration of the inoculum (CFUs) is controlled by quantitative culture. Then, animals are randomly assigned to the different therapeutic regimens, including a control group (infected, no drug). The treatment is usually initiated 18 to 24 hours after bacterial challenge given that the time between i.v. inoculation of the bacteria and start of antimicrobial therapy is critical. As observed in other animal experimental models, this factor can influence the efficacy of tested drugs. Administration of antibiotics is widely realized by the intramuscular (thigh) or i.v. (marginal ear vein) routes. The animals are euthanized by using an i.v. bolus of thiopental at the beginning of the treatment period (controls) or at the end of therapeutic regimen (range, 1 to 5 days). Aortic valve vegetations are excised; immediately placed on ice; and then weighed, homogenized in saline buffer, and plated on agar plates for surviving bacteria counts. Dilutions are used to eliminate potential carryover. Viable counts after 24 h to 48 h of incubation at 37°C are expressed as the mean ± standard deviation log_{10}CFU per gram of vegetation (most reliable judgement criteria). To determine whether antibiotic regimens could induce the selection of in vivo resistant variants, undiluted vegetation homogenates are spread on agar plates containing antibiotic at concentrations corresponding to two- and fourfold the MIC.

The experimental model of endocarditis has demonstrated to be highly valuable in assessing in vivo efficacy of antimicrobial agents by providing endpoints relevant in the evaluation of antibiotics (Lefort & Fantin, 1999):

- Surviving bacteria (expressed as number of CFU per gram of vegetation)
- Blood cultures (positive/negative)
- Ease of removing blood samples (PK assessment)
- Detection of the emergence of resistant variants during therapy
- Mortality
- Incidence of relapse after therapy discontinuation.

3. Linezolid, the first drug issued from the oxazolidinones, a novel class of synthetic antimicrobials

First marketed as oxazolidinone in the early 2000's, linezolid was approved by the United States FDA for the treatment of adults with nosocomial pneumonia, infections due to vancomycin-resistant *Enterococcus faecium*, complicated and uncomplicated skin and skin-structure infections, and community-acquired pneumonia (Zyvox [package insert], 2000). This new drug was considered a promising new option against MRSA in a context of increasing numbers of infections caused by resistant gram-positive bacteria and the emergence of MRSA strains with reduced susceptibility to glycopeptides (Hiramatsu et al., 1997).

3.1 *In vitro* antibacterial activity of linezolid alone and in combination with other antibacterial agents

Oxazolidinones are bacterial protein synthesis inhibitors: linezolid binds to a site on the bacterial 23S ribosomal RNA of the 50S subunit and prevents the formation of a functional 70S initiation complex (Aoki et al., 2002). This mechanism of action is specific to this class, and no cross-resistance with other antimicrobial agents has been observed. As with most protein synthesis inhibitors, linezolid displays nonbactericidal, time-dependent activity in vitro against staphylococci (Kaatz & Seo, 1996) (Figure 1). The bacteriostatic and time-dependent activity did not work in linezolid's favor for clinical use, especially for treatment of severe infections, where most clinicians are convinced that bactericidal drugs are required. Consequently, many studies examined the in vitro activity of linezolid in combination with partner drugs (Table 1), including vancomycin (Grohs et al., 2003; Jacqueline et al., 2003; Soriano et al., 2005; Sahuquillo Arce et al., 2006; Singh et al., 2009), gentamicin (Grohs et al., 2003; Jacqueline et al., 2003), rifampicin (Grohs et al., 2003; Jacqueline et al., 2003; Soriano et al., 2005; Sahuquillo Arce et al., 2006), carbapenems (Jacqueline, 2005, 2006), fosfomycin (Sahuquillo Arce et al., 2006), doxycycline (Sahuquillo Arce et al., 2006), ciprofloxacin (Grohs et al., 2003), levofloxacin (Soriano et al., 2005;

Sahuquillo Arce et al., 2006), and fusidic acid (Grohs et al., 2003). Although indifference is often observed for linezolid combinations against *S. aureus* (including methicillin-resistant strains), some cases of antagonism and synergism were reported and studied in vivo using the experimental model of endocarditis.

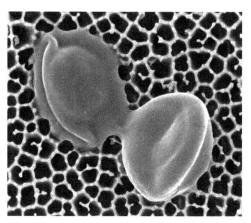

Fig. 1. Scanning electron micrographs of *S. aureus* exposed to linezolid (LNZ) at 8 times the minimum inhibitory concentration (MIC; magnification, ×50,000)

Partner drugs	Class of antibiotics	Interaction	Reference(s)
Vancomycin	Glycopeptides	Antagonism	Grohs et al., 2003; Jacqueline et al., 2003; Soriano et al., 2005; Sahuquillo Arce et al., 2006; Singh et al., 2009;
Gentamicin	Aminoglycosides	Antagonism (inhibition of the early bactericidal activity)	Grohs et al., 2003; Jacqueline et al., 2003
Rifampicin	Rifamycins	Indifference	Grohs et al., 2003; Jacqueline et al., 2003; Soriano et al., 2005; Sahuquillo Arce et al., 2006
Doxycycline	Tetracyclines	Addition	Sahuquillo Arce et al., 2006
Ciprofloxacin	Quinolones	Indifference or Antagonism	Grohs et al., 2003
Levofloxacin			Soriano et al., 2005; Sahuquillo Arce et al., 2006
Acid fusidic	-		Grohs et al., 2003
Fosfomycin	-	Synergy	Sahuquillo Arce et al., 2006
Imipenem	Carbapenems	Synergy	Jacqueline et al., 2005
Ertapenem			Jacqueline et al., 2006

Table 1. In vitro activity of linezolid in combination with partner drugs

3.2 *In vivo* antibacterial activity of linezolid alone and in combination in the experimental model of infective endocarditis

3.2.1 *In vivo* experimental assessment of linezolid activity: Bacteriostatic agent *in vivo*?

First reports of linezolid in vivo activity used oral administration (p.o.) of the drug. Given that linezolid can be administered intravenously (i.v.) or orally, and no dose adjustment is necessary when switching from the i.v. to the oral route of administration in humans (Zyvox [package insert], 2000). Infective endocarditis is considered to require maintenance of bactericidal levels of antibacterial agents for prolonged periods of time to result in eradication of the pathogen. For this reason, it was of special interest to assess the activity of the oxazolidinone in this model of endocarditis. Dailey et al investigated the activity of linezolid at three different p.o. dosages (25, 50, and 75 mg/kg) against MRSA in rabbits with experimental aortic-valve endocarditis (Dailey et al., 2001). After 5 days of treatment, linezolid displayed a stepwise decrease in the mean bacterial counts from the valve vegetation with a significant decrease for both 50 and 75 mg/kg. Showing a 4- to 5-log reduction in valvular bacterial counts, linezolid acted as a bactericidal drug in this study (Dailey et al., 2001).

Based on these results, the authors suggested that linezolid levels at or above the MIC in plasma combined with a minimum number of treatment days was required for the therapeutic efficacy of linezolid in this model. Further studies were then necessary to address the predictive pharmacokinetic and pharmacodynamic (PK/PD) parameters of linezolid.

The extrapolation of results obtained in animal experimental models to human therapy is always a difficult task. Owing to the very short spontaneous half-life of linezolid in rabbits (30 min; unpublished data) and to the difference in bioavailability of orally administered linezolid (approximately 30% bioavailability in rabbits compared to almost 100% in humans (Dailey et al., 2001)), the use of simulation of human pharmacokinetics was required to reach conclusions relevant to human applications. Simulation is particularly suitable for pharmacokinetic and pharmacodynamic analysis, and for the optimization of therapeutic efficacy. Computer-controlled simulation (Bugnon et al., 1998) of human kinetic profiles of linezolid in rabbits was used in the following study to improve the analysis (Jacqueline et al., 2002). The use of a computer-controlled pump allowing an adequate flow of antibiotics to be infused into rabbits enabled us to simulate the in vivo human pharmacokinetics of the antibiotics. The flow can be adjusted to a profile mathematically defined in time (Bugnon et al., 1998). Using this method, the serum linezolid levels obtained after administration of a dose simulating a 10-mg/kg dose in humans are shown in Figure 2. The corresponding mean peak concentration, area under the curve, and half-life were 11.9±1.1 mg/L, 76.3±5.9 mg.h/L, and 2.7±0.1 h, respectively, after administration of the first dose and 21.5±1.3 mg/L, 152.1±9.2 mg.h/L, and 3.4±0.7 h, respectively, at day 5. The increase of linezolid concentrations in plasma at day 5 compared to day 1 suggested drug accumulation as previously shown by Dailey (Dailey et al., 2001) using the same experimental model.

Using the computer-controlled simulation, linezolid significantly decreased the bacterial counts in aortic valve vegetations from rabbits, but failed to exhibit bactericidal activity, despite 5 days of treatment (Figure 3). The comparison with vancomycin administered as a constant-rate intravenous infusion (to obtain a serum steady-state concentration of approximately 20 to 25 mg/L) was in favor of the glycopeptide with at least a 5-$\log_{10}$ colony-forming unit (CFU)/g of vegetation decrease (Figure 3). The oxazolidinone is a time-dependent antibiotic and for these drugs, the time above the MIC (T>MIC) is usually considered a critical parameter in the assessment of therapeutic efficacy (Carbon, 1990). In general, the maximal activity of continuous infusion was obtained at a steady-state concentration in serum equal to a multiple of the MIC, as previously demonstrated for ceftazidime (Cappelletty et al., 1995). To confirm this, continuous infusion of linezolid was used by Jacqueline et al (Jacqueline et al., 2002) to investigate whether it improves in vivo activity. A switch from intermittent dosing to continuous infusion (using the same total daily dose) improved the in vivo activity of linezolid against two strains of MRSA. By increasing the time above the MIC (T>MIC of 100%), linezolid continuous infusion achieved bactericidal activity in vivo with a >3-$\log_{10}$-decrease as compared to the control animals (Figure 4).

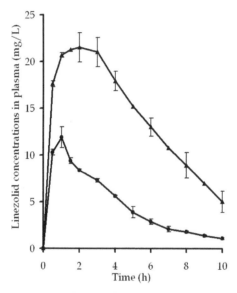

Fig. 2. Linezolid concentrations in plasma after simulation of a dose corresponding to a 10 mg/kg dose in humans (i.e., 600 mg). Circles, concentrations obtained after administration of the first dose; Triangles, concentrations obtained at day 5. Error bars represent standard deviations (adapted from Jacqueline et al., 2002)

Further studies are needed to investigate the potential clinical benefit of continuous infusion, which could be an appropriate alternative to the use of glycopeptides for the treatment of severe MRSA infections. Although no superiority of continuous infusion vs. intermittent dosing was demonstrated in a clinical study with critically ill septic patients (Adembri et al., 2008), Adembri et al showed that the continuous infusion modality has a theoretical advantage over intermittent infusion in the treatment of infection in these patients. Finally, there is a clear need for more powerful clinical trials to demonstrate the potent clinical benefit and the safety of this administration modality.

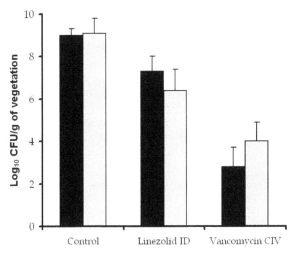

Fig. 3. In vivo activity of linezolid (human-equivalent of 600 mg q12hr, intermittent dosing, ID) and vancomycin (continuous infusion, CIV) against MRSA 1 (black) and MRSA 2 (grey) strains after a 5-day treatment. Error bars represent standard deviations (adapted from Jacqueline et al., 2002)

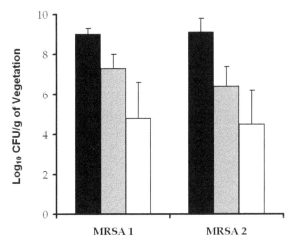

Fig. 4. Impact of the administration mode (intermittent dosing, ID vs. continuous infusion, CIV) on the in vivo activity of linezolid. Control animals (black); Linezolid ID (grey); Linezolid CIV (white). Error bars represent standard deviations (adapted from Jacqueline et al., 2002)

3.2.2 Improvement of the in vivo activity of linezolid by adding a partner drug: What is the good choice?

Infective endocarditis is considered to require bactericidal drugs to achieve clinical efficacy and/or microbiological eradication. Like most protein synthesis inhibitors, oxazolidinones are bacteriostatic agents. Clinicians need to combine linezolid with another drug to (i) increase the bactericidal activity of therapy, (ii) prevent the emergence of drug-resistant subpopulations, and (iii) provide a complementary antibacterial spectrum. Moreover, the use of synergistic antibiotic combinations is appealing as a way to optimize therapy for infective endocarditis, especially when the causative pathogen is resistant (such as MRSA). Although in vitro interactions between linezolid and agents are well-documented (Table 1), the presence of in vitro synergism or antagonism and in vivo correlation or enhanced clinical outcome is not easy to highlight. In addition, the in vitro-in vivo correlation of either positive or negative interactions between two drugs can be difficult to assess and discrepancies occur.

3.2.2.1 Linezolid plus vancomycin

Although the combination of linezolid with vancomycin is not the most obvious choice, many papers have investigated the in vitro activity of this combination and have concluded they are antagonistic. Using the endocarditis model, Chiang et al have tested this association against an MRSA strain and they demonstrated that vancomycin alone was more effective than either linezolid alone or the combination of linezolid and vancomycin (Figure 5) (Chiang & Climo, 2003). This study is in line with in vitro reports (Grohs et al., 2003; Jacqueline et al., 2003) and the combination of linezolid plus vancomycin should be avoided in clinical practice.

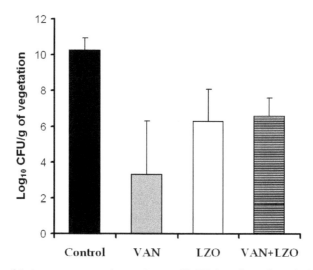

Fig. 5. Outcome of 5-day treatment of experimental MRSA endocarditis. (adapted from Chiang & Climo, 2003)

3.2.2.2 Linezolid plus gentamicin

Linezolid, when added to gentamicin, seemed to inhibit the early in vitro bactericidal activity of gentamicin, particularly over the first 6 h (Jacqueline et al., 2003). During this interval, inhibition of the bactericidal activity of gentamicin was dependent on the linezolid concentration. Aminoglycosides are bactericidal, concentration-dependent antibiotics that act by creating fissures in the outer membrane of the bacterial cell (Gonzalez & Spencer, 1998). A combination of these agents with linezolid could be useful to increase the bactericidal activity of the therapy, especially during the first days of treatment.

Given that the presence of in vitro antagonism is not always correlated with in vivo failure, Jacqueline et al assessed the combination of linezolid plus gentamicin in the endocarditis model against two clinical strains of MRSA exhibiting MICs of 0.125 and 0.5 mg/L (Jacqueline et al., 2004). Using a human-like pharmacokinetic simulation for linezolid and gentamicin, the combination demonstrated a bactericidal activity against the two strains with a decrease of at least 4 $\log_{10}$ CFU/g of vegetation compared with controls. PK/PD aspects could probably explain the difference observed between the in vitro and in vivo activities. Contrary to constant concentrations in time-kill curves experiments, the concentrations of linezolid and gentamicin added to the vegetation changed over time. Although previous in vitro results suggest an antagonism, linezolid combined with gentamicin could be of clinical interest for the treatment of severe MRSA infections requiring combination antimicrobial therapy.

3.2.2.3 Linezolid plus rifampicin

Rifampicin is an RNA polymerase inhibitor that blocks bacterial transcription. Rifampicin is used clinically only as a part of combination regimens because development of resistance is rapid (Heep et al., 2000). In addition to its use against *Mycobacterium tuberculosis*, rifampicin is very useful in the management of bone and joint infections due to MRSA. Indifference was the main interaction observed in vitro between linezolid and rifampicin (Grohs et al., 2003; Jacqueline et al., 2003, Soriano et al., 2005; Sahuquillo Arce et al., 2006). The addition of linezolid prevented the selection of rifampicin resistant mutants after 24 h of incubation at 37°C. Consequently, a synergistic interaction can be considered by inhibition of the emergence of the resistance development.

By evaluating the bactericidal activity, synergy, and emergence of antimicrobial resistance, Dailey et al assessed the potent activity of linezolid plus rifampicin in the endocarditis model against a MSSA strain (rifampicin MIC<= 0.12 mg/L) (Dailey et al., 2003). After a 5-day treatment, the combination showed no in vivo antagonism between the drugs. As with in vitro tests, indifference was observed and the combination inhibited the emergence of rifampicin resistance. These data support a clinical interest in the treatment of infections due to *S. aureus*. A similar study was performed against an MRSA strain (rifampicin MIC= 2 mg/L) and indifference between linezolid and rifampicin was observed (Tsaganos et al., 2008). Moreover, this work demonstrated that (i) linezolid limited bacterial growth in the secondary foci of endocarditis, and (ii) that the combination favored the suppression of bacterial growth in the lung.

3.2.2.4 Linezolid plus carbapenems

Beta-lactam antibiotics act by inhibiting penicillin-binding proteins (PBPs) that are involved in peptidoglycan synthesis. Penicillin-binding protein 2A (PBP2A) is the protein responsible for the methicillin resistance mechanism in *S. aureus*. Methicillin resistance confers resistance to all the beta-lactams, including cephalosporins and carbapenems; however, many studies have reported a potent efficacy of imipenem against *S. aureus* when used in combination with other antimicrobial agents, including fosfomycin (Nakazawa et al., 2003), vancomycin

(Totsuka K et al., 1999; Benquan et al., 2002; Rochon-Edouard et al., 2000), and cephalosporins (Uete & Matsuo et al., 1995).

In vitro synergy between linezolid and carbapenems can be difficult to achieve; sub-inhibitory concentrations of the carbapenem must be used with linezolid to achieve synergy and higher concentrations can lead to an antagonism (Jacqueline, 2005, 2006). The infective endocarditis model was very useful to assess in vivo interaction. Continuous infusion of imipenem alone, the first carbapenem tested in this model, showed no activity against MRSA after 5 days of treatment (Jacqueline et al., 2005). The aim of using continuous imipenem infusion was to obtain an in vivo steady-state concentration that mimics the in vitro conditions so that synergy was observed as soon as possible (i.e., to achieve a target concentration of 1/32 the MIC for each strain). Using these conditions, linezolid plus imipenem exhibited bactericidal and synergistic activities against two MRSA strains, with at least a 4-$\log_{10}$ CFU/g decrease compared to the counts for the controls. Subsequent to that study, the carbapenem ertapenem was investigated in combination with linezolid using the same experimental model (Jacqueline et al., 2006). Ertapenem is a parenteral carbapenem antibiotic with a broad antibacterial spectrum and once-a-day dosing that is supported by clinical studies and an extended half-life (Zhanel et al., 2005). In this study, animals were randomly assigned to receive either no treatment (controls), a linezolid regimen mimicking the human dose of 10 mg/kg/12 h, an ertapenem regimen mimicking the human dose of 1 g/day, or a combination of both regimens. As previously observed with imipenem and confirming the in vitro data, linezolid and ertapenem exhibited a highly bactericidal and synergistic activity in vivo against three MRSA strains after 4 days of treatment (Figure 6). Due to the once-daily dosing of ertapenem and availability of an oral form for linezolid, this combination opens new therapeutic avenues in the field of severe Gram-positive bacterial infections, including an option for outpatient parenteral antimicrobial therapy.

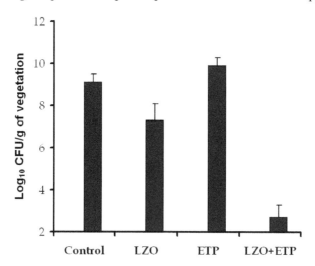

Fig. 6. In vivo synergy between linezolid (LZO) and ertapenem (ETP) against an MRSA strain in the endocarditis model. Error bars represent standard deviations (adapted from Jacqueline et al., 2006)

4. Quinupristin-dalfopristin: A therapeutic option for MRSA endocarditis?

Streptogramins inhibit protein synthesis by binding to the ribosomal 50S subunit, and the most frequent mechanism of quinupristin resistance encountered is target modification by methylation of an adenine residue in 23S rRNA (encoded by the *ermA*, *ermB*, or *ermC* gene). Constitutively expressed *erm* genes confer in vitro cross-resistance to macrolides, lincosamides, and streptogramin B. Quinupristin and dalfopristin are water-soluble injectable streptogramin B and streptogramin A antibiotics, respectively, whose combination in a 30:70 (wt/wt) ratio acts synergistically on Gram-positive bacteria (Bouanchaud, 1992). Despite in vitro susceptibility to quinupristin-dalfopristin, mutations in the L22 ribosomal protein are correlated with resistance to quinupristin in *S. aureus* (Bruni et al., 2000). The experimental model of infective endocarditis was used to address the efficacy of quinupristin-dalfopristin against susceptible and resistant *S. aureus* strains to quinupristin (but not quinupristin-dalfopristin). If quinupristin-dalfopristin remained active against quinupristin-susceptible MRSA after 4 days of treatment, a significant decrease of the activity was observed against a quinupristin-resistant strain. Nevertheless, the impact of the resistance on the activity of the combination can differ between studies (Batard et al., 2002; Pavie et al., 2002).

Combination with vancomycin improved the in vivo activity for susceptible and resistant strains (Pavie et al., 2002), but the benefit was less important against the resistant MRSA. Despite clinical interest in adding gentamicin (aminoglycosides) to quinupristin-dalfopristin, the combination showed no additive benefit against two MRSA strains (Batard et al., 2002). Although the lack of benefit may be due to the high efficacy of the monotherapies, these data did not argue for its use in clinical practice.

5. Daptomycin: Experimental evaluation of an old new drug

Daptomycin, previously called LY 146032, was first discovered in the 1980s by researchers at Eli Lilly, but an increase in creatine phosphokinase levels in serum in early clinical trials (probably related to skeletal muscle toxicity) led to initial abandonment of this promising compound (Tally & DeBruin, 2000).

Daptomycin is a novel lipopeptide antibiotic active against Gram-positive bacteria, including MRSA strains. It disrupts the bacterial cell membrane by forming transmembrane channels, and causes a calcium-dependent depolarization of the cellular membrane and inhibition of macromolecular synthesis leading to cell death (Silverman et al., 2003).

Daptomycin is a potential alternative to vancomycin for the treatment of severe MRSA infections, with benefits such as once-daily dosing, the lack of need for monitoring serum concentrations, and FDA approval for the treatment of right-sided endocarditis (Cubist, 2003). In vitro, the lipopeptide exerts its bactericidal action in a rapid (60 min) and concentration dependent way exhibiting more powerful activity than glycopeptides.

5.1 *In vivo* antibacterial activity of daptomycin: More bactericidal than glycopeptides?

The endocarditis model was used to assess the activity of daptomycin against MRSA and to confirm the highly bactericidal activity observed in vitro, especially in comparison with the reference drug, vancomycin. Effectiveness against three MRSA strains, including one GISA strain (MU50), was tested using computer-controlled simulation to mimic the human dose of 6 mg/kg once daily (Jacqueline et al., 2011). After 4 days of treatment, daptomycin performed well against MSSA, MRSA, and GISA strains (daptomycin MIC= 0.5 mg/L) with a decrease of 5 $\log_{10}$ CFU/g (Figure 7).

More than 20 years ago, Kennedy & Chambers evaluated the potent in vivo activity of daptomycin, known at that time as a vancomycin-like lipopeptide, against *S. aureus* (Kennedy & Chambers, 1989). Vancomycin (25 mg/kg twice daily) was as effective as daptomycin (once-daily dose of 10 mg/kg) against both MSSA and MRSA strains in the endocarditis model. The next year Kaatz et al compared daptomycin (8 mg/kg q8hr) with the glycopeptides, vancomycin and teicoplanin (Kaatz et al., 1990). The conclusion of the study was interesting:

"We have established that, in the rabbit model and against the *S. aureus* test strains we used, daptomycin and teicoplanin-HD are as efficacious as vancomycin, but for certain strains of *S. aureus*, diminished susceptibility to both can develop during therapy" (Kaatz et al., 1990). Also at that time, the authors highlighted an important characteristic of daptomycin, its rapid propensity to select resistant variants during therapy. Despite high in vivo bactericidal activity, experimental models were not able to demonstrate that the rapid bactericidal activity of daptomycin observed in vitro was correlated with a better outcome in vivo than glycopeptides, vancomycin, or teicoplanin.

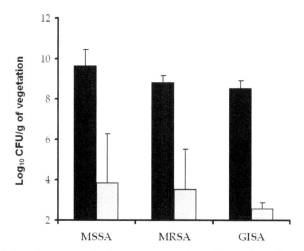

Fig. 7. In vivo activity of daptomycin (human-equivalent (HE) at 6 mg/kg/24 h) against MSSA, MRSA, and GISA strains after a 4-day treatment. Control animals (black); daptomycin-treated animals (grey). Error bars represent standard deviations (adapted from Jacqueline et al., 2011)

5.2 Emergence of daptomycin-resistance during therapy

The experimental endocarditis model is not considered an appropriate model for detection of the emergence of resistant variants. Nevertheless, emergence of daptomycin-resistant variants was observed after only 4 days of therapy in a model using human-equivalent dosage (Jacqueline et al., 2011), as previously shown by Kaatz et al (Kaatz et al., 1990). This strongly suggests that combination therapy may be useful for daptomycin treatment of *S. aureus* infections. In the study by Jacqueline et al, the 6 mg/kg dosage regimen did not prevent the emergence of resistance in two animals (one in the MSSA group (8 animals) and one in the MRSA group (7 animals)) (Figure 8). Moreover, detection of resistant variants was correlated with a failure of daptomycin treatment in those animals. These data support the use of daptomycin dosages exceeding 6 mg/kg to increase bacterial killing and limit the risk of emergence of resistant variants during daptomycin therapy. Case reports have described safe and well tolerated daptomycin treatment at doses up to 12 mg/kg (Benvenuto et al., 2006; Cunha et al., 2006), but adequate dosing of daptomycin remains unresolved. A recent review about clinical utility of daptomycin in infective endocarditis specifies that adequate dosing of daptomycin for the treatment of left-sided or prosthetic valve S. aureus endocarditis should be ≥ 10 mg/kg/day (Cervera et al., 2011).

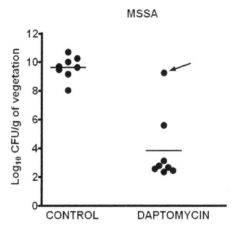

Fig. 8. Bacterial titers in vegetations infected by methicillin-susceptible *S. aureus* after 4 days of treatment with daptomycin (human-equivalent of 6 mg/kg once-daily). Arrows indicate animals with isolates exhibiting increased MICs to daptomycin (adapted from Jacqueline et al., 2011)

5.3 What partner drugs to use with daptomycin? An unresolved question

Faced with rapid emergence of daptomycin-resistant variants during therapy, clinicians should use a combination to limit the risk of resistance development. Rifampicin and gentamicin are often used in combination with antibacterial agents such as glycopeptides, beta-lactams, or linezolid. Two studies investigated the in vivo activity of daptomycin alone and in combination with rifampicin or gentamicin against different MRSA strains (LaPlante & Woodmansee, 2009; Miró et al., 2009). In experiments simulating human PK for all studied drugs, Miro et al demonstrated that daptomycin plus gentamicin was as effective as daptomycin alone (*P*=0.83). In addition, both were more active than daptomycin plus rifampicin (*P*<0.05) (Miró et al., 2009). Using an in vitro pharmacodynamic infection model with simulated endocardial vegetations, LaPlante & Woodmansee showed that daptomycin monotherapy displayed better activity than daptomycin in combination with rifampicin or gentamicin (LaPlante & Woodmansee, 2009). These experimental data strongly show that the addition of gentamicin or rifampicin does not aid the in vivo activity of daptomycin. In vitro, Miro et al (Miro et al., 2009) showed a synergistic interaction between daptomycin and fosfomycin against MSSA and MRSA. Further in vivo and clinical studies are strongly needed to determine effective combinations for avoiding the emergence of resistance to daptomycin.

6. Tigecycline

Tigecycline is the first clinically-available member of a new class of broad-spectrum antibacterials, the glycylcyclines, which were specifically developed to overcome the two major mechanisms of tetracycline resistance (Zhanel et al., 2004). By binding to the 30S ribosomal subunit, tigecycline blocks the entry of aminoacyl-tRNA into the A site of the ribosome during translation (Slover et al., 2007). Like other protein synthesis inhibitors, the drug is bacteriostatic. Tigecycline is an obvious choice to treat MRSA endocarditis, however its potent in vitro activity against MRSA suggests that it should be used as a last resort.

Few studies have valuated the activity of tigecycline in experimental model of MRSA endocarditis. A study using a rat model of endocarditis showed a dose-effect relationship, with a >2-$\log_{10}$ decrease in bacterial counts with doses greater than 10 mg/kg/day for the course of treatment (Murphy et al., 2000). Using a computer-controlled simulation mimicking the human dose of 100 mg initially, followed by 50 mg twice daily, tigecycline demonstrated a significant and homogeneous activity against MSSA, MRSA, and GISA strains (Jacqueline et al., 2011). Nevertheless, the drug failed to exhibit a bactericidal effect versus the effect of the control treatment, despite 4 days of treatment (reduction, 2-$\log_{10}$ CFU/g compared with the controls) (Figure 9). This moderate activity could be improved

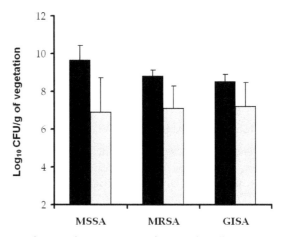

Fig. 9. In vivo outcome after a 4-day treatment of tigecycline (human-equivalent of 100 mg initially, followed by 50 mg twice daily) against MSSA, MRSA, and GISA strains. Control animals (black); tigecycline-treated animals (grey). Error bars represent standard deviations (adapted from Jacqueline et al., 2011)

by the use of a partner drug in combination with tigecycline. The addition of gentamicin significantly improved the killing activity of tigecycline in biofilm-forming *S. aureus* using an in vitro pharmacodynamic model (McConeghy KW & LaPlante, 2010). Finally, studies conducted in both animals and humans have demonstrated that tigecycline distributes widely into various tissues and body fluids (Rello, 2005), and peak serum concentrations do not exceed 1 mg/L, which may limit its utility in the treatment of bacteraemia and endocarditis (Paterson, 2006). The recommended dosage of tigecycline may be too low for the treatment of severe infections and assessment of higher doses in severe experimental animal models is needed.

7. Anti-MRSA cephalosporins exhibiting high affinity for PBP2A: A revolution?

PBPs catalyze transpeptidase or transglycosidase reactions, and are essential for the final stages of peptidoglycan synthesis (Spratt, 1977). β-lactam antibiotics, including penicillins and cephalosporins, inhibit PBPs. β-lactams are widely used because of their broad-spectrum activity and favorable safety profiles (Darville & Yamauchi, 1994). MRSA strains are not susceptible to the action of β-lactams because of the low affinity of β-lactams for PBP2a, an additional PBP encoded by the *mecA* gene and conferring methicillin resistance (Lim & Strynadka, 2002). Because β-lactam antibiotics are usually considered the most effective therapeutic option against *S. aureus* infections, researchers have sought to increase the affinity of β-lactams for the modified PBP2a. This is illustrated by the development of two cephalosporins, namely ceftobiprole and ceftaroline, which have potent antimicrobial activities against both Gram-positive (including MRSA) and Gram-negative bacteria. Ceftaroline binds to the four natural PBPs in *S. aureus*, but has maximum affinity for PBP2a (Villegas-Estrada et al., 2008). Because the marketing authorization for ceftobiprole was withdrawn in the United States and the European Union due to unfavorable assessments of the applications, ceftaroline is better studied.

7.1 Ceftaroline, a broad-spectrum cephalosporin active against MRSA

Ceftaroline is a novel broad-spectrum cephalosporin with potent activity against MRSA strains due to its strong affinity for *S. aureus* PBPs, including PBP2a, encoded by the methicillin resistance gene *mecA* (Lim & Strynadka, 2002). Ceftaroline acetate (PPI-0903) is an N-phosphono-water-soluble prodrug rapidly metabolized in vivo into the bioactive metabolite ceftaroline (PPI-0903 M). In vitro, bactericidal activity (≥ 3 $\log_{10}$ CFU/mL reductions) and time-dependent killing was observed for the cephalosporin from 4 times the MIC against an MRSA strain (Figure 10). Ceftaroline in vivo activity was assessed against two MRSA strains isolated from blood cultures (Jacqueline et al, 2007). The MRSA strain exhibited heterogeneous high-level methicillin resistance (methicillin MIC =128 mg/L), and the heterogeneous glycopeptide- intermediate *S. aureus* strain (hGISA) exhibited homogeneous resistance to methicillin (methicillin MIC >1,024 mg/L) and heterogeneous resistance to glycopeptides. Ceftaroline MICs/MBCs were 1/1 and 2/2 mg/L for the MRSA and hGISA strain, respectively. A human-like simulation was intended to provide apparent values of pharmacokinetic parameters close to those observed in healthy volunteers after a 1-h infusion of a 600-mg dose (approximately 10 mg/kg) of ceftaroline acetate: mean half-life

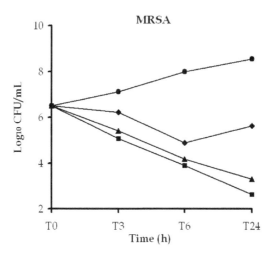

Fig. 10. In vitro activity of ceftaroline against methicillin-resistant *S. aureus*. Control (circles); ceftaroline at 1×MIC (diamonds); ceftaroline at 4×MIC (triangles), ceftaroline at 8×MIC (squares) (Author's unpublished data)

($t1/2$), 1.57 to 2.63 h; peak concentration (Cmax), 18.96 to 21.02 mg/L; and area under the curve (AUC), 56.08 mg.h/L (Cerexa, Inc., unpublished data). After simulation into the rabbit, the corresponding Cmax, AUC, and $t1/2$ values were 21.9±3.0 mg/L, 71.2 mg.h/L, and 2.4 h, respectively (Figure 11). Ceftaroline in vivo activity was assessed against two MRSA strains isolated from blood cultures (Jacqueline et al, 2007). The MRSA strain was a strain with heterogeneous high-level methicillin resistance (methicillin MIC =128 mg/liter), and

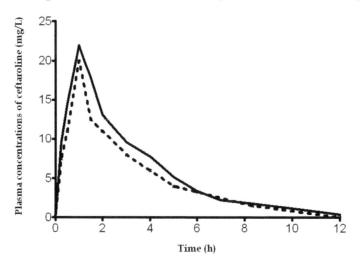

Fig. 11. Pharmacokinetics of ceftaroline in plasma after administration of a dose simulating a 600-mg dose in humans (dashed lines) and the corresponding human pharmacokinetics in animals (solid line) (adapted from Jacqueline et al., 2007)

the heterogeneous glycopeptide- intermediate *S. aureus* strain (hGISA) exhibited homogeneous resistance to methicillin (methicillin MIC >1,024 mg/liter) and heterogeneous resistance to glycopeptides.

Ceftaroline MICs/MBCs were 1/1 and 2/2 mg/L for the MRSA and hGISA strain, respectively. A human-like simulation was intended to provide apparent values of pharmacokinetic parameters close to those observed in healthy volunteers after a 1-h infusion of a 600-mg dose (ca. 10 mg/kg) of ceftaroline acetate: mean half-life ($t1/2$), 1.57 to 2.63 h; peak concentration (Cmax), 18.96 to 21.02 mg/liter; and area under the curve (AUC), 56.08 mg.h/liter (Cerexa, Inc., unpublished data). After simulation into the rabbit, the corresponding Cmax, AUC, and $t1/2$ values were 21.9±3.0 mg/liter, 71.2 mg.h/liter, and 2.4 h, respectively (Figure 11).

In this study, Jacqueline et al evaluated the in vivo activity of ceftaroline in comparison with vancomycin and linezolid, the two main therapeutic options available for the treatment of severe MRSA infections. In vivo outcome after a 4-day treatment is shown in Figure 12. Ceftaroline demonstrated excellent bactericidal and homogeneous activity against MRSA in the endocarditis model with at least a 6-log$_{10}$ CFU/g decrease as compared to the control animals. In comparison, linezolid displayed moderate activity with a 2-log$_{10}$ decrease. Vancomycin was as effective as ceftaroline against the MRSA strain (vancomycin MIC = 1 mg/L), but showed only bacteriostatic activity against the hGISA strain (vancomycin MIC = 4 mg/L). In addition, ceftaroline was able to sterilize 90% and 60% of the vegetations produced by the MRSA or hGISA strain, respectively, whereas vancomycin achieved sterilization of 67% and 0% of the vegetations, respectively.

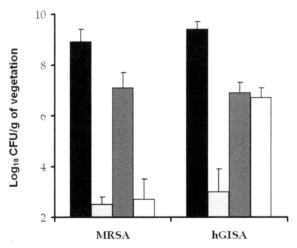

Fig. 12. Bacterial titers in vegetations infected by MRSA or hGISA strains after 4 days of treatment with ceftaroline (human-equivalent of 600 mg twice daily), linezolid (human-equivalent of 600 mg twice daily), and vancomycin (continuous infusion targeting a serum-steady state concentration of 25 mg/L). Control animals (black); ceftaroline-treated animals (grey), linezolid-treated animals (dashed lines), vancomycin-treated animals (white). Error bars represent standard deviations (adapted from Jacqueline et al., 2007)

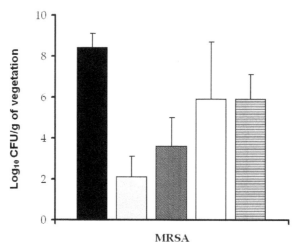

Fig. 13. Bacterial titers in vegetations infected by MRSA after 4 days of treatment with ceftobiprole medocaril (formerly BAL9141) (19 mg/kg of active drug [ceftobiprole] administered intramuscularly thrice daily), daptomycin (intravenous 18 mg/kg once daily), vancomycin (intravenous 30 mg/kg twice daily), and linezolid (75 mg/kg administered subcutaneously three times daily). Control animals (black); ceftaroline-treated animals (grey), linezolid-treated animals (dashed lines), vancomycin-treated animals (white). Error bars represent standard deviations (adapted from Tattevin et al., 2010)

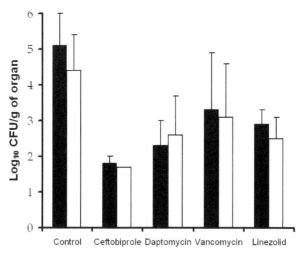

Fig. 14. Bacterial titers in spleens and kidneys after 4 days of treatment with ceftobiprole medocaril (formerly BAL9141) (19 mg/kg of active drug [ceftobiprole] administered intramuscularly thrice daily), daptomycin (intravenous 18 mg/kg once daily), vancomycin (intravenous 30 mg/kg twice daily), and linezolid (75 mg/kg administered subcutaneously three times daily). Spleen bacterial counts (black); Kidney bacterial counts (white). Error bars represent standard deviations (adapted from Tattevin et al., 2010)

Endocarditis studies evaluating the activity of ceftaroline are very limited. However, Tattevin et al have assessed the activity of ceftobiprole (formerly BAL9141), the other anti-MRSA cephalosporin with high affinity for PBP2a, against MRSA in comparison with vancomycin, linezolid, and daptomycin (Tattevin et al, 2010). Using experimental conditions similar to the conditions used by Jacqueline et al, they showed that the burdens of organisms in vegetations were significantly lower in ceftobiprole-treated rabbits than in rabbits treated with vancomycin, linezolid, or daptomycin (4-day treatment) (Figure 13). Moreover, the bacterial titers in spleens and in kidneys were significantly lower in ceftobiprole treated animals than in animals treated by linezolid or vancomycin (Figure 14). A study comparing ceftaroline and daptomycin, and using human-projected doses, demonstrated that both antimicrobial agents displayed highly bactericidal activity against *S. aureus* strains but ceftaroline achieved 100% sterilization of the vegetations infected by the MSSA, MRSA or GISA strains, whereas daptomycin sterilized 62%, 57% and 100% of the vegetations, respectively (Jacqueline et al., 2011).

7.2 Assessment of intramuscular administration of ceftaroline

Pathogens such as MRSA are becoming more virulent and are no longer confined to acute-care settings. There is a clinical need for new antibiotics that can be administered by intramuscular (IM) injection, facilitating outpatient antibiotic therapy for MRSA. The goals of the following experiments were to compare the pharmacokinetic parameters of ceftaroline after intravenous and IM administration and evaluate the in vivo activity of 3 different doses of ceftaroline against MRSA compared with teicoplanin as a positive control after IM administration by using an aortic valve endocarditis rabbit model (Jacqueline et al., 2010).

Six animals were divided into 2 groups, and a 20-mg/kg dose of the prodrug ceftaroline acetate was administered by IM injection into the right thigh or by a short intravenous infusion. Blood samples were obtained from the animals over 8 h (5, 10, 15, 30, and 45 min, and 1, 2, 4, and 8 h post-dose). Results suggest that ceftaroline has an excellent pharmacokinetic profile after IM administration. Bioavailability of IM administration exceeded 90% of intravenous infusion as calculated by AUC (Table 2). C_{max} was decreased with IM administration compared with intravenous infusion as ceftaroline was slowly released from the IM injection site. After IM administration of 5-, 20-, and 40-mg/kg doses, the C_{max} increased approximately in proportion to dose (5.18, 15.75, and 37.85 mg/L, respectively) and plasma half-life increased from 0.74 to 1.14 h (Figure 15). Compared with a short intravenous infusion, IM administration of ceftaroline resulted in longer plasma half-life and percentage of time that the concentration of ceftaroline remained above the MIC (%T>MIC), which is the most critical pharmacokinetic-pharmacodynamic parameter for efficacy (Table 2) (Andes & Craig, 2006).

Using the well-established rabbit endocarditis model, experimental endocarditis was induced with an inoculum of 10^8 CFU of a MRSA strain (ceftaroline MIC = 1 mg/L) with heterogeneous high-level methicillin resistance (methicillin MIC = 128 mg/L). Treatment was started 24 h after inoculation and antibiotics (ceftaroline and teicoplanin) were administered twice daily using the IM route for 4 days. Animals were randomly assigned to no treatment (controls), ceftaroline 40 mg/kg IM twice daily, ceftaroline 20 mg/kg IM twice daily, ceftaroline 5 mg/kg IM twice daily, or teicoplanin 20 mg/kg IM twice daily.

Pharmacokinetic parameter	Ceftaroline 20 mg/kg	
	IM administration	IV administration
C_{max} (mg/L)	16.1 ± 0.7	84.0 ± 7.5
T_{max} (minutes)	30	5
$t_{1/2}$ (hours)	0.9 ± 0.3	0.2 ± 0.00
AUC_{0-8h} (mg•h/L)	26.5 ± 2.9	29.2 ± 3.9
%T>MIC[a] (8-h period)	46.3 ± 2.0	22.5 ± 1.9
%T>MIC[a] (12-h period)	30.9 ± 1.3	15.0 ± 1.3

[a]Methicillin-resistant *Staphylococcus aureus* (MRSA) strain with ceftaroline MIC = 1 mg/L.
AUC = area under the concentration-time curve; C_{max} = peak concentration; T_{max} = time to peak concentration; $t_{1/2}$ = half-life; %T>MIC = time that drug levels in the serum remained above the MIC (Author's unpublished data).

Table 2. Pharmacokinetic parameters following single-dose intramuscular (IM) administration or short intravenous (IV) infusion of ceftaroline (mean ± SD)

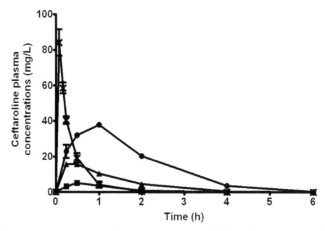

Fig. 15. Ceftaroline concentrations after intramuscular (IM) and intravenous (IV) administration in the rabbit (mean ± SD). ■ = 5-mg/kg IM dose; ▲ = 20-mg/kg IM dose; ● = 40-mg/kg IM dose; × = 20-mg/kg intravenous dose (Author's unpublished data)

The in vivo outcome after a 4-day treatment regimen and the rate of sterilization of the vegetations produced by the MRSA strain are shown in Table 3 (Jacqueline et al., 2010). A dose-dependent response was observed with sterilization rates for ceftaroline of 100%, 80%, and 33% for the 40-mg/kg, 20-mg/kg, and 5-mg/kg doses of ceftaroline, respectively. The difference between 20-mg/kg and 40-mg/kg doses was not statistically significant ($P>0.05$). In vivo bactericidal activity was consistent across all animals tested at the 40-mg/kg dose and for 9 of 10 animals at the 20-mg/kg dose of ceftaroline.

The %T>MICs attained with IM administration in this model were associated with bactericidal activity against MRSA (Tables 2 and 3). The efficacy of IM ceftaroline was similar to that achieved previously with intravenous ceftaroline administered in a regimen simulating the human dose (i.e., 600 mg twice daily) (Jacqueline et al., 2007). As expected, the positive control teicoplanin at 20 mg/kg IM displayed activity against the MRSA strain, with a sterilization rate of 60%, and bacterial titers similar to those observed with vancomycin against the same MRSA strain (Jacqueline et al., 2007). Currently, teicoplanin is the only anti-MRSA drug approved as an IM injection; however, it is not available in the United States. Ceftaroline may be a valuable option for the IM treatment of MRSA infections. These findings are consistent with a favorable IM pharmacokinetic profile and strongly support the development of IM ceftaroline as a promising and effective therapeutic option for the treatment of severe MRSA infections.

Regimen	Mean ± SD $\log_{10}$ CFU/g of vegetation (no. of sterile veg./total no. of veg.) (%)
Controls	8.99 ± 0.47 (0/10) (0)
IM ceftaroline 40 mg/kg	2.45 ± 0.14 (10/10) (100)[a,b,c]
IM ceftaroline 20 mg/kg	3.14 ± 1.38 (8/10) (80)[a,d]
IM ceftaroline 5 mg/kg	5.26 ± 2.73 (3/9) (33)[a]
IM teicoplanin 20 mg/kg	3.07 ± 0.66 (6/10) (60)[a,d]

[a] $P<0.001$ vs controls; [b] $P<0.001$ vs IM ceftaroline 5-mg/kg regimen; Bonferroni's test after analysis of variance. [c] The titers for vegetations from all animals in the group were below the limit of detection. [d] $P<0.05$ vs IM ceftaroline 5-mg/kg regimen. IM = intramuscular.

Table 3. Bacterial titers in vegetations after 4 days of treatment with IM ceftaroline (5, 20, and 40 mg/kg) and IM teicoplanin (20 mg/kg) (adapted from Jacqueline et al., 2010)

8. Conclusions

Antimicrobial therapy is the cornerstone of the treatment of infective endocarditis. Although vancomycin still remains the standard treatment for severe MRSA infections, new therapeutic options are now available for the treatment of MRSA infective endocarditis. Introduction of linezolid, the first member of the oxazolidinone class, in the early 2000s, opened a new field of investigation that demonstrated that vancomycin was not the only solution against MRSA infections. Although linezolid was not the most effective option for endocarditis treatment, studies with the oxazolidinone demonstrated that experimental animal models are essential to (i) develop better understanding of the in vivo activity of a new drug, (ii) obtain important information not present in clinical trials.

Among the new recently available antimicrobial agents, experimental data strongly support daptomycin as an effective option in the treatment of MRSA endocarditis. The lipopeptide demonstrated homogeneous in vivo bactericidal activity against *S. aureus*, including methicillin-susceptible, methicillin-resistant, and glycopeptide-intermediate strains. Taking advantage of favourable drug pharmacokinetics (once-daily administration), daptomycin should be considered as a valuable alternative to vancomycin. Nevertheless, clinical use of daptomycin merit further investigation due to unresolved questions, such as adequate dosing, emergence of resistance during treatment, and appropriate combination therapy.

Ceftaroline fosamil (prodrug of the active metabolite) is a new, broad-spectrum cephalosporin recently approved in the USA for the treatment of acute bacterial skin and skin structure infections and community-acquired bacterial pneumonia. Data from both clinical trials (Corey et al., 2010; Wilcox et al., 2010; Rank et al., 2011) and animal studies confirmed ceftaroline as a very promising new cephalosporin for the treatment of serious MRSA infections. Given its safety profile, bactericidal activity, and excellent activity against *S. aureus*, ceftaroline should play an important role in the treatment of MRSA infective endocarditis in the coming years.

9. References

Adembri, C., Fallani, S., Cassetta, M.I., Arrigucci, S., Ottaviano, A., Pecile, P., Mazzei, T., De Gaudio, R. & Novelli, A. (2008). Linezolid pharmacokinetic/pharmacodynamic profile in critically ill septic patients: intermittent versus continuous infusion. *International Journal of Antimicrobial Agents*, Vol.31, No.2, pp. 122-129.

Andes, D. & Craig, W.A. (2006). Pharmacodynamics of a new cephalosporin, PPI-0903 (TAK-599), active against methicillin-resistant *Staphylococcus aureus* in murine thigh and lung infection models: identification of an *in vivo* pharmacokinetic-pharmacodynamic target. *Antimicrobial Agents and Chemotherapy*, Vol.50, No.4, pp. 1376–1383.

Aoki, H., Ke, L., Poppe, S.M., Poel, T.J., Weaver, E.A., Gadwood, R.C., Thomas, R.C., Shinabarger, D.L. & Ganoza, M.C. (2002). Oxazolidinone antibiotics target the P site on *Escherichia coli* ribosomes. *Antimicrobial Agents and Chemotherapy*, Vol.46, No.4, pp. 1080–1085.

Batard, E., Jacqueline, C., Boutoille, D., Hamel, A., Drugeon, H.B., Asseray, N., Leclercq, R., Caillon, J., Potel, G. & Bugnon, D. (2002). Combination of quinupristin-dalfopristin and gentamicin against methicillin-resistant *Staphylococcus aureus*: Experimental rabbit endocarditis study. *Antimicrobial Agents and Chemotherapy*, Vol.46, No.7, pp. 2174-2178.

Benquan, W., Yingchun, T., Kouxing, Z., Tiantuo, Z., Jiaxing, Z. & Shuqing, T. (2002). *Staphylococcus* heterogeneously resistant to vancomycin in China and antimicrobial activities of imipenem and vancomycin in combination against it. *Journal of Clinical Microbiology*, Vol.40, No.3, pp. 1109-1112.

Benvenuto, M., Benziger, D.P., Yankelev, S. & Vigliani, G. (2006). Pharmacokinetics and tolerability of daptomycin at doses up to 12 milligrams per kilogram of body weight once daily in healthy volunteers. *Antimicrobial Agents and Chemotherapy*, Vol.50, No.10, pp. 3245-3249.

Bouanchaud, D.II. (1992). *In-vitro* and *in-vivo* synergic activity and fractional inhibitory concentration (FIC) of the components of a semisynthetic streptogramin, RP 59500. *Journal of Antimicrobial Chemotherapy*, Vol.30 (Suppl. A), pp. 95–99.

Bugnon, D., Potel, G., Caillon, J., Baron, D., Drugeon, H.B., Feigel, P., Kergueris, M.F. (1998). *In vivo* simulation of human pharmacokinetics in the rabbit. *Bulletin of Mathematical Biology*, Vol.60, No.3, pp. 545-567.

Boucher, H.W., Talbot, G.H., Bradley, J.S., Edwards, J.E., Gilbert, D., Rice, L.B., Scheld, M., Spellberg, B. & Bartlett, J. (2009). Bad bugs, no drugs: no ESKAPE! An update from the Infectious Diseases Society of America. *Clinical Infectious Diseases*, Vol.48, No.1, pp. 1-12.

Carbon, C. (1990). Impact of the antibiotic schedule on efficacy in experimental endocarditis. *Scandinavian Journal of Infectious Diseases*, Suppl. 74, pp. 163–172.

Cappelletty, D.M., Kang, S.L., Palmer, S.M. & Rybak, M.J. (1995). Pharmacodynamics of ceftazidime administered as continuous infusion or intermittent bolus alone and in combination with single daily-dose amikacin against *Pseudomonas aeruginosa* in an *in vitro* infection model. *Antimicrobial Agents and Chemotherapy*, Vol.39, No.8, pp. 1797–1801.

Cervera, C., Castañeda, X., Pericas, J.M., Del Río, A., de la Maria, C.G., Mestres, C., Falces, C., Marco, F., Moreno, A. & Miró, J.M. (2011). Clinical utility of daptomycin in infective endocarditis caused by Gram-positive cocci. *International Journal of Antimicrobial Agents*, [Epub ahead of print].

Chiang, F.Y. & Climo, M. (2003). Efficacy of linezolid alone or in combination with vancomycin for treatment of experimental endocarditis due to methicillin-resistant *Staphylococcus aureus*. *Antimicrobial Agents and Chemotherapy*, Vol.47, No.9, pp. 3002-3004.

Corey, G.R., Wilcox, M.H., Talbot, G.H, Thye, D., Friedland, D., Baculik, T. & CANVAS 1 investigators. (2010). CANVAS 1: the first Phase III, randomized, double-blind study evaluating ceftaroline fosamil for the treatment of patients with complicated skin and skin structure infections. *Journal of Antimicrobial Chemotherapy*, 65 Suppl 4, pp. 41-51.

Cubist Pharmaceuticals. (2003). Cubicin (daptomycin for injection). *Cubist Pharmaceuticals*, Lexington, MA, USA.

Cunha, B.A., Eisenstein, L.E. & Hamid, N.S. (2006). Pacemaker-induced *Staphylococcus aureus* mitral valve acute bacterial endocarditis complicated by persistent bacteremia from a coronary stent: Cure with prolonged/high-dose daptomycin without toxicity. *Heart Lung*, Vol.35, No.3, pp. 207-211.

Dailey, C.F., Dileto-Fang, C.L., Buchanan, L.V., Oramas-Shirey, M.P., Batts, D.H., Ford, C.W. & Gibson, J.K. (2001). Efficacy of linezolid in treatment of experimental endocarditis caused by methicillin-resistant *Staphylococcus aureus*. *Antimicrobial Agents and Chemotherapy*, Vol.45, No.8, pp. 2304-2308.

Dailey, C.F., Pagano, P.J., Buchanan, L.V., Paquette, J.A., Haas, J.V. & Gibson, J.K. (2003). Efficacy of linezolid plus rifampin in an experimental model of methicillin-susceptible *Staphylococcus aureus* endocarditis. *Antimicrobial Agents and Chemotherapy*, Vol.47, No.8, pp. 2655-2658.

Darville, T. & Yamauchi, T. (1994). The cephalosporin antibiotics. *Pediatrics in Review*, Vol.15, No.2, pp. 54-62.

Durack, D.T. & Beeson, P.B. (1972). Experimental bacterial endocarditis. I. Colonization of a sterile vegetation. *British Journal of Experimental Pathology*, Vol.53, No.1, pp. 44-49.

Durack, D.T. & Beeson, P.B. (1972). Experimental bacterial endocarditis. II. Survival of a bacterium in endocardial vegetations. *British Journal of Experimental Pathology*, Vol.53, No.1, pp. 50-53.

Entenza, J.M., Que, Y.A., Vouillamoz, J., Glauser, M.P. & Moreillon P. (2001). Efficacies of moxifloxacin, ciprofloxacin, and vancomycin against experimental endocarditis due to methicillin-resistant *Staphylococcus aureus* expressing various degrees of ciprofloxacin resistance. *Antimicrobial Agents and Chemotherapy*, Vol.45, No.11, pp. 3076-3083.

Fowler, V.G. Jr., Scheld, W.M. & Bayer, A.S. (2005). Endocarditis and intravascular infections, In: *Mandell, Douglas, and Bennett's Principles and Practice of Infectious Diseases, Sixth Edition*, pp. 975–1022, Philadelphia: Elsevier Churchill Livingstone.

Garrison, P.K. & Freedman, L.R. (1970). Experimental endocarditis I. Staphylococcal endocarditis in rabbits resulting from placement of a polyethylene catheter in the right side of the heart. *Yale Journal of Biology and Medicine*, Vol.42, No.6, pp. 394-410.

Gonzalez, L.S. 3rd. & Spencer, J.P. (1998). Aminoglycosides: a practical review. *American Family Physician*, Vol.58, No.8, pp. 1811-1820.

Grohs, P., Kitzis, M.D. & Gutmann, L. (2003). *In vitro* bactericidal activities of linezolid in combination with vancomycin, gentamicin, ciprofloxacin, fusidic acid, and rifampin against *Staphylococcus aureus*. *Antimicrobial Agents and Chemotherapy*, Vol.47, No.1, pp. 418-420.

Heep, M., Rieger, U., Beck, D. & Lehn, N. (2000). Mutations in the beginning of the rpoB gene can induce resistance to rifamycins in both *Helicobacter pylori* and *Mycobacterium tuberculosis*. *Antimicrobial Agents and Chemotherapy*, Vol.44, No.4, pp. 1075-1077.

Hiramatsu, K., Hanaki, H., Ino, T., Yabuta, K., Oguri, T. & Tenover, F. C. (1997). Methicillin-resistant *Staphylococcus aureus* clinical strain with reduced vancomycin susceptibility. *Journal of Antimicrobial Chemotherapy*, Vol.40, No.1, pp. 135–136.

Jacqueline, C., Batard, E., Perez, L., Boutoille, D., Hamel, A., Caillon, J., Kergueris, M.F., Potel, G. & Bugnon, D. (2002). *In vivo* efficacy of continuous infusion versus intermittent dosing of linezolid compared to vancomycin in a methicillin resistant *Staphylococcus aureus* rabbit endocarditis model. *Antimicrobial Agents and Chemotherapy*, Vol.46, No.12, pp. 3706-3712.

Jacqueline, C., Caillon, J., Le Mabecque, V., Miegeville, A.F., Donnio, P.Y., Bugnon, D. & Potel, G. (2003). *In vitro* activity of linezolid alone and in combination with gentamicin, vancomycin or rifampicin against methicillin-resistant *Staphylococcus aureus* by time-kill curve methods. *Journal of Antimicrobial Chemotherapy*, Vol.51, No.4, pp. 857-864.

Jacqueline, C., Asseray, N., Batard, E., Le Mabecque, V., Kergueris, M.F., Dube, L., Bugnon, D., Potel, G. & Caillon, J. (2004). *In vivo* efficacy of linezolid in combination with gentamicin for the treatment of experimental endocarditis due to methicillin-resistant *Staphylococcus aureus*. *International Journal of Antimicrobial Agents*, Vol.24, No.4, pp. 393-396.

Jacqueline, C., Navas, D., Batard, E., Miegeville, A.F., Le Mabecque, V., Kergueris, M.F., Bugnon, D., Potel, G. & Caillon, J. (2005). *In vitro* and *in vivo* synergistic activities of linezolid combined with subinhibitory concentrations of imipenem against methicillin-resistant *Staphylococcus aureus*. *Antimicrobial Agents and Chemotherapy*, Vol.49, No.1, pp. 45-51.

Jacqueline, C., Caillon, J., Grossi, O., Le Mabecque, V., Miegeville, A.F., Bugnon, D., Batard, E. & Potel, G. (2006). *In vitro* and *in vivo* assessment of linezolid combined with ertapenem: a highly synergistic combination against methicillin-resistant *Staphylococcus aureus*. *Antimicrobial Agents and Chemotherapy*, Vol.50, No.7, pp. 2547-2549.

Jacqueline, C., Caillon, J., Le Mabecque, V., Miègeville, A.F., Hamel, A., Bugnon, D., Ge, J.Y. & Potel G. (2007). *In vivo* efficacy of ceftaroline (PPI-0903), a new broad-spectrum cephalosporin, compared with linezolid and vancomycin against methicillin-resistant and vancomycin-intermediate *Staphylococcus aureus* in a rabbit endocarditis model. *Antimicrobial Agents and Chemotherapy*, Vol.51, No.9, pp. 3397-3400.

Jacqueline, C., Caillon, J., Batard, E., Le Mabecque, V., Amador, G., Ge, Y., Biek, D. & Potel, G. (2010). Evaluation of the in vivo efficacy of intramuscularly administered ceftaroline fosamil, a novel cephalosporin, against a methicillin-resistant *Staphylococcus aureus* strain in a rabbit endocarditis model. *Journal of Antimicrobial Chemotherapy*, Vol.65, No.10, pp. 2264-2265.

Jacqueline, C., Amador, G., Batard, E., Le Mabecque, V., Miègeville, A.F., Biek, D., Caillon, J. & Potel G. (2011). Comparison of ceftaroline fosamil, daptomycin and tigecycline in an experimental rabbit endocarditis model caused by methicillin-susceptible, methicillin-resistant and glycopeptide-intermediate *Staphylococcus aureus*. *Journal of Antimicrobial Chemotherapy*, Vol.66, No.4, pp. 863-866.

Kaatz, G.W., Seo, S.M., Reddy, V.N., Bailey, E.M. & Rybak, M.J. (1990). Daptomycin compared with teicoplanin and vancomycin for therapy of experimental *Staphylococcus aureus* endocarditis. *Antimicrobial Agents and Chemotherapy*, Vol.34, No.11, pp. 2081-2085.

Kaatz, G.W. & Seo, S.M. (1996). *In vitro* activities of oxazolidinone compounds U100592 and U100766 against *Staphylococcus aureus* and *Staphylococcus epidermidis*. *Antimicrobial Agents and Chemotherapy*, vol.40, No.3, pp. 799–801.

Kennedy, S. & Chambers, H.F. (1989). Daptomycin (LY146032) for prevention and treatment of experimental aortic valve endocarditis in rabbits. *Antimicrobial Agents and Chemotherapy*, Vol.33, No.9, pp. 1522-1525.

LaPlante, K.L. & Woodmansee, S. (2009). Activities of daptomycin and vancomycin alone and in combination with rifampin and gentamicin against biofilm-forming methicillin-resistant *Staphylococcus aureus* isolates in an experimental model of endocarditis. *Antimicrobial Agents and Chemotherapy*, Vol.53, no.9, pp. 3880-3886.

Lefort, A., & Fantin, B. (1999). Rabbit model of bacterial endocarditis, In: *Handbook of animal models of infection*, O. Zak & M.A. Sande, (Ed.), 611-617, ISBN 0-12-775390-7.

Lim, D. & Strynadka, N.C. (2002). Structural basis for the beta lactam resistance of PBP2a from methicillin-resistant *Staphylococcus aureus*. *Nature Structural Biology*, Vol.9, No.11, pp. 870-876.

McConeghy, K.W. & LaPlante, K.L. (2010). *In vitro* activity of tigecycline in combination with gentamicin against biofilm-forming *Staphylococcus aureus*. *Diagnostic Microbiology and Infectious Disease*, Vol.68, No.1, pp. 1–6.

Malbruny, B.; Canu, A., Bozdogan, B., Zarrouk, V., Fantin, B. & Leclercq, R. (2000). Quinupristin/Dalfopristin resistance Mutation Reveals the Involvement of L22 Ribosomal Protein in Synergy Between Quinupristin and Dalfopristin, *Proceedings of 40th Interscience Conference Antimicrobial Agents and Chemotherapy*, p. 118, Abstr. No. 1928, Toronto, Ontario, Canada, September 17-20, 2000.

Maltezou, H.C. (2009). Metallo-beta-lactamases in Gram-negative bacteria: introducing the era of pan-resistance? *International Journal of Antimicrobial Agents*, Vol.33, No.5, pp. 405-407.

Miró, J.M., García-de-la-Mària, C., Armero, Y., Soy, D., Moreno, A., del Río, A., Almela, M., Sarasa, M., Mestres, C.A., Gatell, J.M., Jiménez de Anta, M.T., Marco, F. & Hospital

Clinic Experimental Endocarditis Study Group. (2009). Addition of gentamicin or rifampin does not enhance the effectiveness of daptomycin in treatment of experimental endocarditis due to methicillin-resistant *Staphylococcus aureus*. *Antimicrobial Agents and Chemotherapy*, Vol.53, No.10, pp. 4172-4177.

Miró, J.M., Entenza, J.M., del Río, A., García-de-la-Mària, C., Giddey, M., Armero, Y., Cervera, C., Mestres, C.A., Almela, M., Falces, C., Marco, F., Moreillon, P. & Moreno, A. (2009). Daptomycin (DAP) plus Fosfomycin (FOM) is Synergistic against Methicillin-Susceptible (MSSA) and Methicillin-Resistant *Staphylococcus aureus* (MRSA) Strains: From Bench to Bedside. *Proceedings of 49th Interscience Conference Antimicrobial Agents and Chemotherapy*, Abstr. No. E-1449, San Francisco, CA, USA, September 12-15, 2009.

Murphy, T.M., Deitz, J.M., Petersen, P.J., Mikels, S.M. & Weiss, W.J. (2000). Therapeutic efficacy of GAR-936, a novel glycylcycline, in a rat model of experimental endocarditis. *Antimicrobial Agents and Chemotherapy*, Vol.44, No.11, pp. 3022-3027.

Nakazawa, H., Kikuchi, Y., Honda, T., Isago, T. & Nozaki, M. (2003). Enhancement of antimicrobial effects of various antibiotics against methicillin-resistant *Staphylococcus aureus* (MRSA) by combination with fosfomycin. *Journal of Infection and Chemotherapy*, Vol.9, No.4, pp. 304-309.

Paterson, D.L. (2006). Clinical experience with recently approved antibiotics. *Current Opinion in Pharmacology*, Vol.6, No.5, pp. 486–490.

Pavie, J., Lefort, A., Zarrouk, V., Chau, F., Garry, L., Leclercq, R. & Fantin, B. (2002). Efficacies of quinupristin-dalfopristin combined with vancomycin *in vitro* and in experimental endocarditis due to methicillin-resistant *Staphylococcus aureus* in relation to cross-resistance to macrolides, lincosamides, and streptogramin B- type antibiotics. *Antimicrobial Agents and Chemotherapy*, Vol.46, No.9, pp. 3061-3064.

Rank, D.R., Friedland, H.D. & Laudano, J.B. (2011). Integrated safety summary of FOCUS 1 and FOCUS 2 trials: Phase III randomized, double-blind studies evaluating ceftaroline fosamil for the treatment of patients with community-acquired pneumonia. *Journal of Antimicrobial Chemother*, 66 Suppl 3, pp. 53-59.

Rello, J. (2005). Pharmacokinetics, pharmacodynamics, safety, and tolerability of tigecycline. *Journal of Chemotherapy*, Vol.17 (Suppl 1), pp. 12–22.

Rochon-Edouard, S., Pestel-Caron, M., Lemeland, J.F. & Caron, F. (2000). *In vitro* synergistic effects of double and triple combinations of beta-lactams, vancomycin, and netilmicin against methicillin-resistant *Staphylococcus aureus* strains. *Antimicrobial Agents and Chemotherapy*, Vol.44, No.11, pp. 3055-3060.

Sahuquillo Arce, J.M., Colombo Gainza, E., Gil Brusola, A., Ortiz Estévez, R., Cantón, E. & Gobernado, M. (2006). *In vitro* activity of linezolid in combination with doxycycline, fosfomycin, levofloxacin, rifampicin and vancomycin against methicillin-susceptible *Staphylococcus aureus*. *Revista Espanola de Quimioterapia*, Vol.19, No.3, pp. 252-257.

Sakoulas, G., Eliopoulos, G.M., Alder, J. & Eliopoulos, C.T. (2003). Efficacy of daptomycin in experimental endocarditis due to methicillin-resistant *Staphylococcus aureus*. *Antimicrobial Agents and Chemotherapy*, Vol.47, No.5, pp. 1714-1718.

Silverman, J.A., Perlmutter, N.G. & Shapiro, H.M. (2003). Correlation of daptomycin bactericidal activity and membrane depolarization in *Staphylococcus aureus*. *Antimicrobial Agents and Chemotherapy*, Vol.47, No.8, pp. 2538-2544.

Singh, S.R., Bacon, A.E. 3rd., Young, D.C. & Couch, K.A. (2009). *In vitro* 24-hour time-kill studies of vancomycin and linezolid in combination versus methicillin-resistant *Staphylococcus aureus*. *Antimicrobial Agents and Chemotherapy*, Vol.53, No.10, pp. 4495-4497.

Slover, C.M., Rodvold, K.A. & Danziger, L.H. (2007). Tigecycline: a novel broad-spectrum antimicrobial. *Annals of Pharmacotherapy*, Vol.41, No.6, pp. 965-972.

Soriano, A., Jurado, A., Marco, F., Almela, M., Ortega, M. & Mensa, J. (2005). *In vitro* activity of linezolid, moxifloxacin, levofloxacin, clindamycin and rifampin, alone and in combination, against *Staphylococcus aureus* and *Staphylococcus epidermidis*. *Revista Espanola de Quimioterapia*, Vol.18, No.2, pp. 168-172.

Spratt, B.G. (1977). Properties of the penicillin binding proteins of *Escherichia coli* K12. *European Journal of Biochemistry*, Vol.72, No.2, pp. 342-352.

Tally, F.P. & DeBruin, M.F. (2000). Development of daptomycin for Gram-positive infections. *Journal of Antimicrobial Chemotherapy*, Vol.46, No.4, pp. 523–526.

Tattevin, P., Basuino, L., Bauer, D., Diep, B.A. & Chambers, H.F. (2010). Ceftobiprole is superior to vancomycin, daptomycin, and linezolid for treatment of experimental endocarditis in rabbits caused by methicillin-resistant *Staphylococcus aureus*. *Antimicrobial Agents and Chemotherapy*, Vol.54, No.2, pp. 610-613.

The 10 x '20 Initiative: pursuing a global commitment to develop 10 new antibacterial drugs by 2020. (2010). Infectious Diseases Society of America. *Clinical Infectious Diseases*, Vol.50, No.8, pp. 1081-1083.

Totsuka, K., Shiseki, M., Kikuchi, K. & Matsui, Y. (1999). Combined effects of vancomycin and imipenem against methicillin-resistant *Staphylococcus aureus* (MRSA) *in vitro* and *in vivo*. *Journal of Antimicrobial Chemotherapy*, Vol.44, No.4, pp. 455-460.

Tsaganos, T., Skiadas, I., Koutoukas, P., Adamis, T., Baxevanos, N., Tzepi, I., Pelekanou, A., Giamarellos-Bourboulis, E.J., Giamarellou, H. & Kanellakopoulou, K. (2008). Efficacy and pharmacodynamics of linezolid, alone and in combination with rifampicin, in an experimental model of methicillin-resistant *Staphylococcus aureus* endocarditis. *Journal of Antimicrobial Chemotherapy*, Vol.62, No.2, pp. 381-383.

The bacterial challenge: time to react, In: European Centre for Disease Prevention and Control, European Medicines Agency Joint Technical report, September 2009, Available from
http://www.emea.europa.eu/pdfs/human/antimicrobial resistance.

Uete, T. & Matsuo, K. (1995). Synergistic enhancement of *in vitro* antimicrobial activity of imipenem and cefazolin, cephalothin, cefotiam, cefamandole or cefoperazone in combination against methicillin-sensitive and -resistant *Staphylococcus aureus*. *Japanese Journal of Antibiotics*, Vol.48, No.3, pp. 402-408.

Villegas-Estrada, A., Lee, M., Hesek, D., Vakulenko, S.B. & Mobashery, S. (2008). Co-opting the cell wall in fighting methicillin-resistant *Staphylococcus aureus*: potent inhibition of PBP 2a by two anti-MRSA beta-lactam antibiotics. *Journal of the American Chemical Society*, Vol.130, No.29, pp. 9212-9213.

Wilcox, M.H., Corey, G.R., Talbot, G.H., Thye, D., Friedland, D., Baculik, T. & CANVAS 2 investigators. (2010). CANVAS 2: the second Phase III, randomized, double-blind study evaluating ceftaroline fosamil for the treatment of patients with complicated skin and skin structure infections. *Journal of Antimicrobial Chemotherapy*, 65 Suppl 4, pp. 53-65.

Zak, O., Sande, M., & O'Reilly, T. (1999). Introduction: the role of animal models in the evaluation of new antibiotics, In: *Handbook of animal models of infection*, O. Zak & M.A. Sande, (Ed.), 611-617, ISBN 0-12-775390-7.

Zhanel, G.G., Homenuik, K., Nichol, K., Noreddin, A., Vercaigne, L., Embil, J., Gin, A., Karlowsky, J.A. & Hoban, D.J. (2004). The glycylcyclines: a comparative review with the tetracyclines. *Drugs*, Vol.64, No.1, pp. 63-88.

Zhanel, G.G., Johanson, C., Embil, J.M., Noreddin, A., Gin, A., Vercaigne, L. & Hoban, D.J. (2005). Ertapenem: review of a new carbapenem. *Expert Review of Anti-Infective Therapy*, Vol.3, No.1, pp. 23-39.

Zyvox [package insert]. (2000). *Pharmacia & Upjohn Company*, Kalamazoo, MI, USA.

6

NVS and Staphylococci in the Oral Cavity – A Cause of Infective Endocarditis

Yuko Ohara-Nemoto[1], Shigenobu Kimura[2] and Takayuki K. Nemoto[1]
*[1]Department of Oral Molecular Biology, Course of Medical and Dental Sciences,
Nagasaki University Graduate School of Biomedical Sciences
[2]Division of Molecular Microbiology, Department of Microbiology,
Iwate Medical University
Japan*

1. Introduction

Oral streptococci including viridans streptococci and nutritionally-variant streptococci (NVS) along with *Staphylococcus* species including *Staphylococcus aureus* and coagulase negative staphylococci (CoNS) are two main bacterial groups known to be causative of infective endocarditis (IE). These bacteria are not pathogenic in principal for healthy individuals, and streptococci are regular commensal occupants of the oral microflora as well as the gastrointestinal tract and female genital tract. *Staphylococcus* species also comprise normal human microflora of the skin, nasal cavity, and gastrointestinal tract. The infectious routes for these pathogenic bacteria entering the bloodstream are not identified in half of examined IE patients. In addition to oral streptococci, *staphylococcus* species are generally isolated from dental plaque and saliva (Smith et al., 2001; Ohara-Nemoto et al., 2008a), thus the oral cavity is considered to be a common habitat for the two main pathogenic bacteria of IE. These findings suggest that peroral bacterial transmission to the bloodstream should be examined as a cause of IE, while systematic studies of the relationships between IE and oral conditions, such as extent of periodontal disease, dentate state (dentate, edentulous, denture wearing), and oral hygiene, are also needed to elucidate the causative role of oral bacteria. From the point of disease due to peroral bacteremia, it is of interest that a substantial part of staphylococcal arthritis is considered to originate from the oral cavity (Jackson et al., 1999). This review focuses on causative bacteria of IE that mainly colonize the oral cavity and their pathogenicity.

2. Causative bacteria of infective endocarditis

IE, an infection of the endocardium of the heart, is an uncommon but life-threatening disease with a high mortality rate ranging from 10-24% (Ferreiros et al., 2006; Yoshinaga et al., 2008; Murdoch et al., 2009). The overall incidence rate has been found to range from 4.4 to 11.6 cases per 100,000 person-years (Berlin et al., 1995; Tleyjeh et al., 2005; Fedeli et al., 2011). Cardiac valvular abnormalities that cause eddy- or jet-type vascular flow are strong risk factors (Strom et al., 1998; Nakatani et al., 2003). Abnormal vascular flow around valves causes clotting deposits, and bacteria which enter the bloodstream and become attached to clots then grow by forming biofilm. According to the most recent surveillance data (848 IE cases reported in 2000 and 2001), the characteristics of IE in Japan include mean age of 55±18 years, with most patients aged from 50 to 70 years, with 82% of IE patients complicated with underlying diseases, such as valvular heart disease (65%), congenital heart disease (9%), or particular implantation (3%), whereas in 18% cases IE occurred without any predisposing cardiac diseases (Nakatani et al., 2003). Noticeably, a route of infection was not identified in 53.9% of those cases. Also, patients with etiologically unidentified IE had no prior infectious disease causing bacteremia, such as urinary tract infection, pneumonia, or cellulitis, and no history of invasive procedure or intravenous drug administration. Thus, it is considered especially important to identify the infectious routes of etiologically unidentified IE in Japan.

The second most common etiology in Japanese IE cases was found to be post-dental procedures and oral hygiene-related conditions in those with viridans streptococci infection (35.7%). Viridans streptococci, indigenous bacteria in the oral cavity, are most frequently identified as pathogenic bacteria of IE and in Guidelines presented in 2003 by the Japanese Circulation Society it was noted that dental procedures may cause IE. This medical background in Japan may be different from Western countries, because no link between IE and dental treatment was shown in a population-based case-control study performed in the United States (Strom et al., 1998).

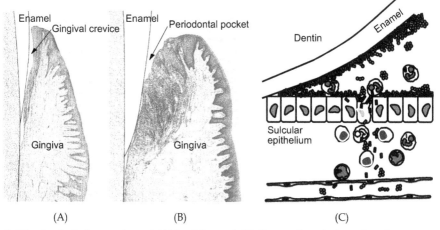

(A)   (B)   (C)

Fig. 1. Histological observation of (A) healthy and (B) diseased periodontal regions. (C) Scheme of dentogingival junction. The periodontal crevice is bathed in the gingival crevicular fluid. In periodontal disease, a crevice becomes a pocket. Polymorphonuclear neutrophils migrate to the crevice, and lymphocytes and monocytes are shown in a connective tissue. Oral microorganisms are expected to enter into the bloodstream through gingival sulcular epithelium and connective tissue

Until recently, viridans streptococci have been considered as the most common causative microorganisms of IE and detected at a range from 30% to 50% (Strom et al., 1998; Nakatani et al., 2003; Murdoch et al., 2004; Tleyjeh et al., 2005; Alshammary et al., 2008). Viridans streptococci are composed of a total of 21 species, including *S. mitis, S. anginosus, S. salivalius,* and *S. bovis* (Kawamura et al., 1995). Because of their non-pathogenicity in principal and phenotypical characteristic resemblance, clinical isolates of viridans streptococci obtained from patients with various diseases are usually not identified at the bacterial species level, but rather registered as '*Streptococcus viridans*' or viridans streptococci. For these, though *S. sanguinis* and *S. oralis* are considered to be the most common agents of streptococcal IE, information is limited and molecular based-species identification is needed to clarify their pathogenicity.

In addition to frequent isolation of viridans streptococci, a finding that edentulous state decreased IE risk (Strom et al., 2000) suggests that the opportunity for transmission and amount of transmitting bacteria through the dentogingival interface are functionally important issues in regard to onset of the disease (Okell et al., 1935; Carmona et al., 2002; Ohara-Nemoto et al., 2008a).

Following the incidence rate of IE by viridans streptococci, infection by *Staphylococcus aureus* is significant and ranges from 17% to 43%, while that in combination with CoNS ranges from 9% to 13%. The changing spectrum from streptococci to staphylococci has been reported in recent epidemiological studies performed in many countries (Sandre & Shafran, 1996; Hoen et al., 2002; Cecchi et al., 2004, Ferreiros et al., 2006; Alshammary et al., 2008; Fedeli et al., 2011). *S. aureus* has also been identified as a leading cause of death cases (Alshammary, et al., 2008; Yoshinaga et al., 2008). Etiologic *Staphylococcus* spp. causing IE are assumed to be acquired via a percutaneous route from skin flora, especially in nosocomial infection cases and intravenous drug abusers. However, its infectious route is often not described in cases in Japan (Niwa et al., 2005) and France (Di Filippo et al., 2006). With this in mind, it is reasonable to speculate that a part of staphylococcal IE is caused by peroral infection as in IE cases with viridans streptococci, because the occurrence of oral staphylococci is significantly higher than generally accepted. For example, the prevalence rate of *Staphylococcus* species was found to be 73% in dental plaque and 84% in saliva (Ohara-Nemoto et al., 2008a). In accordance with the existence of oral staphylococci, Etienne et al. (1986) reported cases of staphylococcal IE resulting from dental extraction.

Microorganisms are not found in approximately 15% of the IE cases in Japan, a part of which might be related to NVS, because NVS organisms scarcely grow in ordinary growth media, and require an L-cysteine or pyridoxal supplement. *Abiotrophia defectiva*, formerly *Streptococcus defectiva*, was first described as a new type of viridans group of streptococci 50 years ago (Frenkel & Hirsch, 1961). Later, according to 16S rRNA sequence findings, the genus *Abiotrophia* as well as genus *Granulicatella* was taxonomically established from NVS (Collins & Lawson, 2000). The genus *Abiotrophia* is composed of one species of *A. defectiva*, while the genus *Granulicatella* is composed of *G. adiacens* and *G. elegans*, which are isolated from humans, and *G. balaenopterae* from minke whales. Most clinical strains of NVS reported were isolated as agents of subacute IE and accounted for more than 4% of streptococcal IE (Bouvet, 1995). NVS are also constituents of the normal flora of the oral cavity and upper respiratory tract (George, 1974, Ruoff, 1991, Ohara-Nemoto et al., 1997), thus the infection route for NVS causing IE is likely peroral.

3. NVS

3.1 Occurrence and molecular identification of NVS in saliva and dental plaque specimens

NVS do not grow on Trypticase soy agar with 5% sheep blood, which can support growth of viridans streptococci, whereas they usually grow on either chocolate or Burucella agar with 5% horse blood (Ruoff, 2007), or in nutritionally rich broth supplemented with L-cysteine or pyridoxal (Fenkel & Hirsch, 1961). Furthermore, NVS generally grow well in medium from a commercially available culture bottle system for anaerobic bacteria, such as BACTEC PLUS Anaerobic/F culture bottles at 37°C under anaerobic conditions (Ohara-Nemoto et al., 2005).

To isolate NVS from oral or combined infection specimens, a culture method for monitoring the bacteriolytic activity of NVS may be useful. This activity toward *Micrococcus luteus* was demonstrated only with NVS species and not with other viridans streptococci isolated from IE cases or oral bacteria (Pompei et al., 1990). Using this method, we isolated NVS from saliva and dental plaque specimens (Ohara-Nemoto et al., 1997). Briefly, after appropriate dilutions with phosphate-buffered saline, oral specimens were inoculated onto a double-layer nutrient agar plate with a top layer containing heat-killed *M. luteus* ATCC 9341 and cultured overnight. Use of an anaerobic condition raised the growth rate of NVS as compared with the aerobic condition. Isolates exhibiting bacteriolytic activity, shown as a colony surrounded with a clear halo, were NVS. These isolates also demonstrated satellitism with a streak of *S. aureus* on a Todd-Hewitt agar plate. For species identification, molecular based methods, i.e., 16S rRNA sequencing or 16S rRNA PCR followed by restriction fragment length polymorphism analysis (PCR-RFLP) (Ohara-Nemoto et al., 1997; Ohara-Nemoto et al., 2005), were successfully applied. When 92 oral NVS strains were examined, the PCR-RFLP patterns of *G. adiacens* and *A. defectiva* were readily distinguished from each other, as well as from those of other streptococcal and enterococcal species (Fig. 2).

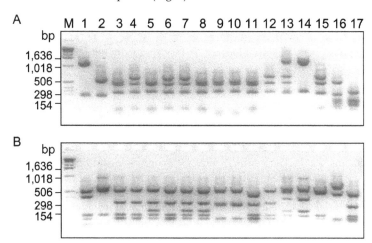

Fig. 2. 16S rDNA PCR-RFLP of *G. adiacens*, *A. defectiva*, and viridans streptococci. The 16S rRNA gene (1.5 kb) was amplified by PCR using a set of universal primers for eubacteria, then cleaved with (A) *Hae*III or (B) *Msp*I. Lanes: M, size marker; 1, *G. adiacens*; 2, *A. defectiva*; 3, *sanguinis*; 4, *S. oralis*; 5, *S. gordonii*; 6, *S. mitis*; 7, *S. salivarius*; 8, *S. bovis*; 9, *S. mutans*; 10, *S. sobrinus*; 11, *S. pyogenes*; 12, *S. pneumoniae*; 13, *S. aureus*; 14, *S. epidermidis*; 15, *Enterococcus faecalis*; 16, *Haemophilus influenzae*; 17, *Escherichia coli*

Species identification performed by PCR-RFLP completely matched that obtained by phenotypic characteristics. Consequently, it was found that the occurrence of NVS in dental plaque and saliva specimens from healthy dental students was relatively high, as 97.8%

(91/93) of the subjects harbored either one of the two bacterial species. In addition, the prevalence of *G. adiacens* was 87.1% and that of *A. defectiva* was 11.8%, which were comparable or even higher than those of viridans streptococci (Kimura & Ohara-Nemoto, 2007). Interestingly, except for one subject carrying both species, all carried only one, suggesting that these two species may be incompatible with each other.

Recently, Shimoyama et al. (2011) developed a rapid and highly sensitive 16S rRNA PCR identification method for NVS using species-specific sets of primers. With this method, *G. adiacens* (including *G. para-adjacens*) was detected in most healthy adult subjects, followed by *A. defectiva* and *G. elegans* (unpublished results). The high level of occurrence of NVS in the oral cavity demonstrated by this and previous reports (Ohara-Nemoto et al., 1997; Sato et al., 1999) is in good agreement with recent results of normal oral flora examined from 5 subjects ranging in age from 23 to 55 years old (Aas et al., 2005). A culture-independent 16S rRNA gene cloning and sequencing method demonstrated that *S. mitis* and related species were most commonly found in all sites of the oral cavity, followed by the two *Granulicatella* species. *G. adiacens* and *G. elegans* were commonly detected in most areas, such as the buccal, vestibule, tongue dorsum, tongue lateral, hard palate, soft palate, tonsils, tooth surface, and subgingival sites in a wide range of ages. Although the detection rate of *A. defectiva* was somewhat lower than that of *Granulicatella* species, this bacterium was also among the top 21 of commonly observed bacteria of 141 predominant species in the oral cavity. Therefore, with the high occurrence of NVS in the oral cavity in mind, a relatively high incidence of NVS-related IE (more than 4% of streptococcal IE) may be reasonable. Elucidation of the prevalence rates and amounts of NVS in the oral cavity, especially in elderly subjects whose incidence rate for IE is remarkably high, may contribute to better understanding of the pathological process of NVS-related IE. Non-culture methods targeting 16S rRNA (Goldenberger et al., 1997; Shimoyama et al., 2011) are convenient and practical for this purpose.

3.2 Cases of IE caused by NVS

Most clinical NVS isolates reported were derived from culturing blood obtained from IE patients and up to 100 cases of NVS IE have been presented to date. We treated an IE case with severe mitral and aortic valves insufficiencies caused by *G. elegans* derived from the oral cavity (Ohara-Nemoto et al., 2005). A 53-year-old previously healthy female without anamnesis had undergone a dental procedure at a local clinic two months before consulting with us. The patient had a slight fever and cough, and was diagnosed with chronic heart failure and transferred to an outside facility, where IE associated with aortic and mitral valve vegetation was noted in echocardiography findings. Four consecutive arterial and venous blood cultures were successively performed at other and our facilities with BACTEK PLUS Anaerobic/F culture bottles and Brucella HK agar plates under anaerobic conditions. Two sets of cultures were positive and yielded gram-positive coccoides in short chains. At our hospital, the patient received antibiotic treatment with intravenous benzylpenicillin (1.2 million units per day) and gentamicin (60 mg per day), then cardiac surgery was performed 7 days after admission. The left coronary cups of the aortic valve showed perforation and ulceration with multiple vegetation sites, and the mitral valve anterior leaflets were perforated with large amounts of vegetation. The patient was released from the hospital without a fever after 27 days.

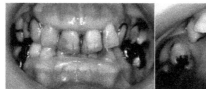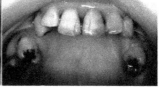

Fig. 3. Oral findings of a patient with IE caused by *G. elegans*. Dental plaque was collected from right upper |34 (Ohara-Nemoto et al., 2005)

Bacterial isolates from the patient were identified as *G. elegans* (IMU02b01) by microbiological characteristics and 16S rRNA gene sequencing. An oral examination of the patient one week after surgery showed widespread redness of the gingiva, dental caries, and deposition of a large amount of dental plaque (Fig. 3). The oral state of the patient suggested a risk of bacteremia due to increased dentogingival surface area, with oral *G. elegans* the suspected agent in this case.

Characteristic	Result for *G. elegans* strain[a]:		
	IMU02b01	IMU02p18	CCUG 26024
Enzyme production	+	+	+
Pyrrolidonyl aminopeptidase	-	-	-
Alkaline phosphatase	-	-	-
Urease	+	+	+
Arginine dihydrolase	-	-	-
α-Galactosidase	-	-	-
β-Galactosidase	-	-	-
β-Glucuronidase	+	+	+
α-Glucosidase	-	-	-
β-Glucosidase	+	+	+
Hippurate hydrolysis	-	-	-
Acetoin production	-	-	-
Acidification of:			
Trehalose	-	-	-
Lactose	-	-	-
Raffinose	-	-	-
Sucrose	+	+	+
Melibiose	-	-	-
Arabinose	-	-	-
Sorbitol	-	-	-
Mannitol	-	-	-
Growth in THB supplemented with:			
L-Cysteine HCL (0.01 %)	+	+	+
Pyridoxal HCL (0.001 %)	-	-	-

[a] +, positive result; -, negative result

Table 1. Biochemical characteristics of blood- and oral cavity-derived *G. elegans* isolates from an IE patient

To confirm our speculation, a *G. elegans* strain was isolated from a dental plaque specimen obtained from the patient using a selective culture method. As a result, strain IMU03p18 was obtained, which exhibited the same basic phenotypic characteristics as strains IMU02b01 and *G. elegans* CCUG 26024 (Table 1) (Roggenkamp et al., 1998). Among these characteristics, urease production, acidification of raffinose and sucrose, and hydrolysis of hippurate have been reported to be strain dependent (Roggenkamp et al., 1998; Sato et al., 1999; Collins et al., 2000).

We found that both IMU02p18 and IMU02b01 were negative for urease, positive for hippurate hydrolysis, and fermented sucrose but not raffinose. In addition, their antimicrobial susceptibility tendencies were identical, as they were highly susceptible to penicillin and other β-lactams, whereas they were intermediate to amikacin and resistant to arbekacin (Table 2). These properties were in accordance with other *G. elegans* isolates from IE patients (Ruoff, 1991; Tuohy et al., 2000). In accordance with observed in vitro antibiotic susceptibility, combination treatment with benzylpenicillin and gentamicin was effective in this case. Pulsed-field gel electrophoresis (PFGE) and arbitrarily primed PCR also demonstrated that the genotypes of the two strains isolated from blood and dental plaque samples obtained from the patient were indistinguishable from each other (Fig. 4). These phenotypical and molecular-based characteristics clearly indicated that they were derived from an identical clone. Thus, our findings suggested peroral infection of *G. elegans* in this case of IE.

Agent	MIC (µg/ml) [a]		
	IMU02b01	IMU02p18	CCUG 26024
Penicillin	≤0.06	≤0.06	≤0.06
Ampicillin	≤0.25	≤0.25	≤0.25
Cefazolin	≤0.5	≤0.5	≤0.5
Ceftazidime	≤0.5	≤0.5	≤0.5
Cefozopran	≤0.5	≤0.5	≤0.5
Cefdinir	≤0.12	≤0.12	≤0.12
Cefepime	≤0.12	≤0.12	≤0.12
Imipenem	≤0.12	≤0.12	≤0.12
Gentamicin	≤4	≤4	≤4
Amikacin	32	32	≤16
Arbekacin	>16	>16	≤4
Erythromycin	≤0.25	≤0.25	≤0.25
Clarithromycin	≤0.25	≤0.25	≤0.25
Clindamycin	≤0.25	≤0.25	≤0.25
Minocycline	≤2	≤2	≤2
Vancomycin	1	1	≤0.5
Teicoplanin	≤1	≤1	≤1
Fosfomycin	16	16	16
Levofloxacin	≤2	≤2	≤2
Sulfamethoxazole-Trimethoprim	40	40	40

Table 2. Antimicrobial susceptibility of blood- and oral cavity-derived *G. elegans* isolated from an IE patient. [a]MICs were determined using a micro-dilution method developed by the National Committee for Clinical Laboratory Standards

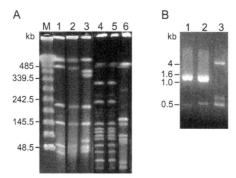

Fig. 4. Molecular based identification of *G. elegans* isolates from blood culture and dental plaque of the IE patient. (A) PFGE was performed after digestion with *Sma*I (lanes 1 to 3) and *Apa*I (lanes 4 to 6). Lanes: M, DNA markers; 1 and 4, IMU02b01; 2 and 5, IMU02p18; 3 and 6, *G. elegans* CCUG 26024. (B) Arbitrarily primed-PCR. Lanes: 1, IMU02b01; 2, IMU02p18; 3, *G. elegans* CCUG 26024

4. Staphylococci

4.1 Occurrence of staphylococci in the oral cavity

Staphylococcus species involving *S. aureus* are considered to be transient bacteria in the oral cavity and the amounts of these organisms in oral specimens (10^2-10^4 cfu/ml in saliva, 10^3-10^5 cfu/g in dental plaque) are quite low as compared to those of viridans streptococci (10^4-10^6 cfu/ml in saliva, 10^7-10^9 cfu/g in dental plaque). However, it is evident that *Staphylococcus* species, especially *S. epidermidis* and *S. aureus*, are frequently isolated from the oral cavity (Reviewed by Smith et al., 2001; El-Solh et al., 2004; Murdoch et al., 2004; Ohara-Nemoto et al., 2008a). Interestingly, oral staphylococcal possession in adults aged from 20 to over 80 years old ranges from 60% to 88%, with the highest prevalence (88% in saliva) observed with elderly subjects aged from 60 to 79 years (Percival et al., 1991). Furthermore, the prevalence of staphylococci at sites of periodontal disease (59%) was found to be significantly higher than that of healthy subgingival sites: 54% in diseased sites and 29% in periodontally healthy control sites (Murdoch et al., 2004).

In addition to dental interest, oral staphylococci have been suggested to be an infectious source of rheumatoid arthritis. Staphylococci are the most common causes of bacterial arthritis in adults, among which *S. aureus* is the primary agent (Goldenberg, 1998; Ryan et al., 1997). Similar to etiologically unidentified cases of IE, etiological sources are not identified in up to 30% of bacterial arthritis cases (Kaandorp et al., 1997). Thus, it is speculated that oral microflora plays a role in the reservoir of agents related to staphylococcal arthritis. According to the report by Jackson et al. (1999), the occurrence of oral staphylococci was 94% in healthy adults (mean 32 years old) and that in healthy elderly subjects (mean 82 years old) was 100%, with 36% of those elderly subjects found to be colonized by *S. aureus*. Furthermore, in rheumatoid arthritis patients (mean 60 years old), staphylococci were isolated from 96% and the proportion of subjects with oral *S. aureus* was 56%, which was significantly higher than that of the healthy subjects (24%). Jacobson et al. (1997) also demonstrated a higher prevalence of *S. aureus* isolated from the oral cavity of patients with rheumatoid arthritis. These findings are of particular interest when considering cases of etiologically unidentified staphylococcal IE.

Our previous study of the occurrence of oral staphylococci also aimed to identify a potential peroral route of staphylococcal IE (Ohara-Nemoto et al., 2008a). *Staphylococcus species* were isolated from saliva and supragingival dental plaque specimens obtained from systemically and dentally healthy adults (n=56, mean 27.1±5.3 years old) using a culture method. Consequently, along with 99 *S. aureus* isolates and 235 isolates of *S. intermedius* and CoNS species, at least 9 of 15 *Staphylococcus* species known to colonize in humans were observed in the oral cavity (Table 3). The isolation frequencies of staphylococci were 83.9% in saliva and 73.2% in dental plaque. Furthermore, *S. epidermidis* (60.7%) and *S. aureus* (46.4%) were the species most frequently isolated from plaque and saliva, respectively, followed in order by *S. hominis, S. warneri, S. intermedius, S. capitis,* and *S. haemolyticus* (12.5-7.1%) from both locations. In contrast, *S. gallinarum* and *S. lugdunensis* were rarely isolated (1/56, 1.8% of all cases) (Table 3). The prevalence tendency of oral staphylococci was similar to that of specimens obtained from the nasal cavity. Staphylococci-positive subjects (n=47) harbored from 1 to 5 species (mean 2.3±1.0) (a portion of those results is shown in Table 4). In addition to *S. aureus* and *S. epidermidis, S. capitis, S. hominis, S. lugdunensis,* and *S. warneri* have been implicated in IE.

Species	No. of positive subjects (% isolation frequency)		
	Saliva[a]	Plaque[a]	Nasal swab[b]
S. aureus	26 (46.4)	19 (33.9)	8 (44.4)
S. capitis	5 (8.9)	5 (8.9)	3 (16.7)
S. epidermidis	23 (41.1)	34 (60.7)	13 (72.2)
S. gallinarum	1 (1.8)	0 (0)	0 (0)
S. haemolyticus	4 (7.1)	3 (5.4)	1 (5.6)
S. hominis	7 (12.5)	7 (12.5)	4 (22.2)
S. intermedius	5 (8.9)	5 (8.9)	1 (5.6)
S. lugdunensis	1 (1.8)	0 (0)	0 (0)
S. warneri	6 (10.7)	5 (8.9)	3 (16.7)
Total staphylococci	47 (83.9)	41 (73.2)	17 (94.4)

Table 3. Occurrence of staphylococci in saliva, dental plaque, and nasal samples. [a]None of the subjects had received antibiotic medication within the previous 3 months (n=56, aged 22-43 years old, 27.1±5.3 years; 37 males, 19 females). [b]Nasal swab samples were taken from 18 (32.7±2.6 years: 12 males, 6 females) of 47 oral staphylococci-positive subjects

The genetic relatedness of these staphylococcal isolates was examined by PFGE and the results revealed nasal-oral trafficking of *Staphylococcus* species (Fig. 5), as PFGE patterns indicated that clinical staphylococcal isolates from each subject were identical clones or close relatives. Furthermore, a longitudinal examination over a 2-month period demonstrated that a single identical or same combination of *Staphylococcus* species was continuously isolated. Thus, *Staphylococcus* species found in the oral cavity are regular residential composers of oral microflora or may be continuously provided from the nasal cavity.

Subject no.	Saliva	Plaque	Nasal
1	***S. aureus***	***S. aureus***	***S. aureus***, *S. epidermidis, S. hominis*
2	***S. aureus, S. epidermidis***, *S. hominis*	*S. aureus, S. epidermidis, S. hominis*	***S. aureus***
3	***S. aureus***, *S. intermedius*	***S. aureus***	***S. aureus***, *S. warneri*
4	***S. aureus***, *S. warneri*	***S. aureus, S. epidermidis***	***S. aureus***, *S. capitis,* ***S. epidermidis***
5	***S. aureus, S. epidermidis***	*S. intermedius*	***S. aureus, S. epidermidis***
6	***S. epidermidis***	***S. aureus, S. epidermidis***	***S. aureus, S. epidermidis***, *S. hominis*
7	*S. aureus,* ***S. epidermidis***	***S. epidermidis***	***S. epidermidis***
8	***S. epidermidis***	***S. epidermidis***	***S. epidermidis***
9	***S. epidermidis***	***S. epidermidis***, *S. capitis, S. haemolyticus*	***S. epidermidis***
10	***S. epidermidis***, *S. hominis, S. warneri*	***S. epidermidis***, *S. intermedius*	***S. epidermidis***, *S. capitis, S. hominis*
11	*S. aureus,* ***S. lugdunensis***	*S. aureus,* ***S. epidermidis***, *S. warneri*	***S. epidermidis, S. lugdunensis***
12	*S. aureus, S. warneri*	***S. epidermidis***	***S. epidermidis***
13	*S. capitis*	***S. hominis***	***S. hominis***, *S. warneri*
14	*S. epidermidis*	*S. epidermidis*	*S. capitis, S. hominis*
15	*S. capitis*	ND	*S. aureus, S. epidermidis, S. warneri*
16	*S. epidermidis*	*S. epidermidis*	ND
17	*S. intermedius, S. warneri*	*S. warneri*	*S. aureus, S. epidermidis*
18	*S. intermedius*	ND	*S. epidermidis*

Table 4. Staphylococcal species isolated from oral and nasal cavities. Genetic relatedness of the isolates in bold was confirmed by PFGE. ND, not detected

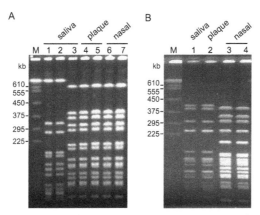

Fig. 5. Genetic relatedness of oral and nasal *S. aureus* (A) or *S. epidermidis* (B) isolates obtained from subjects No. 1 and No. 7 in Table 4, respectively Chromosomal DNA of isolates from oral and nasal specimens was digested with *Sma*I, then separated using PFGE. The relative coefficients of the strains examined were 100% (A, lanes 3-7) and 82.7% (B, lanes 1-4)

Although the composition and proportions of oral microflora in adults are rather stable over long periods, it is notable that occurrence rates of staphylococci, mainly *S. aureus*, tend to increase with age, which is possibly associated with xerostomia (decrease in saliva flow) and denture wearing. The occurrence of staphylococci (88%) was found to be significantly high in denture plaque (Marsh & Martin, 2009), presumably because of their capability of adherence to prosthetic materials. Similarly, *S. aureus* and *S. epidermidis* are the most common pathogens isolated from disease sites of late prosthetic joint infections (Maderazo et al., 1988). On the other hand, the occurrence rates of *S. mutans* and other viridans streptococci are consistent over time after tooth eruption (Percival et al., 1991). This event may be explained by the finding that *S. mutans* colonizes the tongue coat of elderly individuals after loss of teeth, while the prevalence of *Porphyromonas gingivalis*, a major agent of chronic periodontitis, was shown to be closely related to the presence of teeth with periodontal pockets (Kishi et al., 2010). Therefore, when considering that IE as well as rheumatoid arthritis is age-related disease, we speculate that microflora of dental plaque and possibly denture plaque serve to harbor *Staphylococcus* species that cause these diseases. Oral staphylococci are more important for high-risk IE subjects when they are dentate (presence of dentogingival interface) and have poor oral hygiene. Furthermore, periodontal diseases may increase the risk of staphylococcal bacteremia due to increases in dentogingival surface area and bacterial numbers of *S. aureus*. Notably, a recent study also reported a correlation between staphylococci from the oral cavity and developments of atherosclerosis and cardiovascular diseases (Koren et al., 2011).

4.2 Pathogenicity factors of staphylococci

4.2.1 Biofilm formation

A biofilm is a multi-layered membranous aggregate of microorganisms attached to a biotic or abiotic surface. Oral bacteria that colonize on tooth surfaces and soft epithelial tissues are considered to grow primarily based on their ability to form biofilm, as this attachment system is necessary to prevent evacuation by host swallowing. *Staphylococcus* and *Streptococcus* species including NVS form biofilms. For all these except *S. aureus*, which produces potent virulence factors, their ability of biofilm formation plays a role as a major virulence factor of IE. Biofilm components include self-produced polymeric matrix and adhesins, which mediate the primary attachment of bacteria to endocardium and heart valve surfaces, followed by intercellular adhesion. Bacteria in biofilm resist host defenses and antibiotic treatment. Numerous studies have demonstrated that biofilms consist of 4 principal factors; teichoic acids, polysaccharide intercellular adhesins such as PIA from *S. epidermidis* or PNAG from *S. aureus*, extracellular DNA (ecDNA), and proteinaceous adhesins.

Teichoic acid is a cell wall component of gram-positive bacteria, and recently found to be an essential constituent of staphylococcal biofilms (Gross et al., 2001; Sadovskaya et al., 2005). Cell wall and extracellular teichoic acids are a mixture of two kinds of polymers, $\alpha(1\rightarrow5)$-linked poly(ribitol phosphate), substituted at the 4-position of ribitol residues with β-GlucNAc, and $(1\rightarrow3)$-linked poly(glycerol phosphate), partially substituted with D-Ala at the 2-position of glycerol residue (Vinogradov et al., 2006). Since a large fraction of teichoic acid is located in the 'fluffy'-layer region beyond the cell wall, it is considered that it functions in primary adhesion of bacteria to attached surfaces.

The glucosamine-based extracellular polysaccharides PIA and PNAG (PIA/PNAG) is an identical chemical compound, poly-$\beta(1,6)$-N-acetyl-D-glucosamine, which is responsible for cell-cell attachment (Mack et al., 1996; Cramton et al., 1999). PIA/PNAG is synthesized by enzymes encoded by the *icaADBC* (intercellular adhesin) operon (Heilmann et al., 1996; Götz, 2002) and *icaADBC* mutants of *S. epidermidis* RP62A were shown not to form biofilm (Gerke et al., 1998). However, it has also been demonstrated with many clinical isolates that PIA/PNAG-negative *S. epidermidis* and *S. aureus* exhibit a strong biofilm phenotype (Rohde et al., 2007; Hennig et al., 2007; Boles et al., 2010). Rohde et al. (2007) reported that 27% of biofilm-positive *S. epidermidis* isolates produced PIA-independent biofilms, some of which were possibly mediated by the proteinaceous adhesin Aap, an accumulation-associated protein (Hussain et al., 1997). In addition, other proteins, such as the cell wall lytic enzyme AtlE (Heilmann et al., 1996), biofilm-associated protein Bap (Cucarella et al., 2001), and others are involved in attachment to the polymer surface or host matrix proteins, and related to cell-cell adhesion (Frank & Patel, 2007; Otto, 2009).

It was recently shown that AtlE is responsible for autolysis of *S. epidermidis*, resulting in release of ecDNA, and that ecDNA is a structural component of biofilms formed by *S. epidermidis* and *S. aureus* (Qin et al., 2007; Rice et al., 2007). The ratios of these 3 factors, PIA/PNAG, proteinous, and ecDNA, in biofilm formation seem to be varied for each strain, and become altered by various environmental or culture conditions. The ratios were conveniently semi-quantified *in vitro* by measuring amounts of biofilms formed on polymeric surfaces after incubation with or without dispersin B, trypsin, and DNaseI (Izano et al., 2008). We observed that production of the major extracellular protease GluSE was enhanced under specific culture conditions that also increased biofilm formation (Fig. 6) (Ohara-Nemoto et al., 2002). This observation is quite interesting with considering the relationship to a recent finding that protein-dependent biofilm formation by *S. aureus* was inhibited by expressions of extracellular proteases (Martí et al., 2010). The involvement of proteases in staphylococcal and streptococcal biofilm formation remains to be clarified.

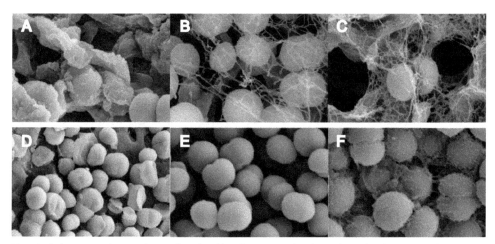

Fig. 6. Culture condition-dependent biofilm formation by *S. epidermidis*. Scanning electron micrographs of 'biofilm-negative' *S. epidermidis* ATCC 12228 (A and D) and 14990 (B and E), and 'biofilm-positive' ATCC 35984 (C and F). Bacteria were cultured in Todd-Hewitt broth (THB) agar (A-C) or THB (D-F). Biofilm formation was clearly demonstrated with strains 12228 and 14990 cultured on THB agar, while it was not evident when these were cultured in THB

4.2.2 Staphylococcal glutamic acid-specific protease

Glutamic acid-specific staphylococcal GluV8-family proteases belong to a serine protease family that possesses a catalytic triad composed of Ser, Asp, and His, forming a competent electron relay. GluV8 from *S. aureus*, first reported by Drapeau et al. (1972) as V8 protease, is related to its bacterial growth *in vivo* and pathogenicity (Coulter et al., 1998). GluV8 processes adhesion molecules that are expressed on the bacterial cell surface and destroy the extracellular matrix of host cells (Karlsson & Arvidson, 2002). GluSE was found as an *S. epidermidis* GluV8 homolog, which is the most abundant extracellular protein (Sasaki et al., 1998), and efficiently degrades host proteins such as elastin, fibronectin, collagen, complement protein C5, and immunoglobulin (Dubin et al., 2001; Moon et al., 2001; Ohara-Nemoto et al., 2002). The gene encoding GluSE is ubiquitously distributed on the chromosome and the protein is expressed in most clinical isolates under *in vitro* culture conditions (Fig. 7). Production frequency was comparable between isolates from patients suffering from IE,

1 2   3 4   5 6 7 8 9 10 11 12 13

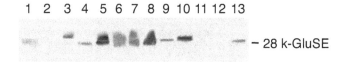

− 28 k-GluSE

Fig. 7. GluSE production in *S. epidermidis* clinical isolates. Extracellular soluble fractions were subjected to SDS-polyacrylamide gel electrophoresis, followed by immunoblotting with anti-GluSE Ig. Lanes 1-6, isolates from patients: lanes 7-12, isolates from saliva of healthy individuals: 13, purified GluSE

bacteremia, and wound infection (7/10, 70%), as well as in saliva from healthy subjects (44/59, 74.6%) (Ikeda et al., 2004).

As demonstrated by 2D-PAGE followed by protein identification with MALDI TOF-MS and immunoblotting, 28-kDa mature GluSE was observed as the major extracellular protein constituent (Fig. 8A), while another Glu-specific cysteine proteinase, Ecp, was moderately expressed (Ohara-Nemoto et al., 2008b). In a cell wall fraction, limited amounts of 32-, 30-, and 29-kDa proforms of GluSE were observed (Fig. 8B and C), whereas no pro- or matureforms of GluSE were detected in bacterial cytoplasm. These findings indicated that GluSE is immediately secreted after protein synthesis and maturation through cleavage at the Ser_{-1}-Val_1 bond.

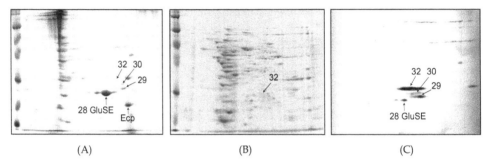

(A) (B) (C)

Fig. 8. 2D-PAGE shows GluSE in extracellular and cell wall fractions. The extracellular fraction of *S. epidermidis* (A) and cell wall fractions (B and C) were separated by 2D-PAGE, and developed with Coomassie brilliant blue staining (A and B) or immunoblotting with anti-GluSE Ig (C). Numbers indicate relative molecular weights (kDa)

Genes encoding GluV8 homologs were recently cloned from other CoNS species, and their proteolytic activities and biochemical characteristics were determined (Nemoto et al., 2008; Ono et al., 2010): They are GluSW from *S. warneri*, GluScp from *S. caprae*, and GluScoh from *S. cohnii*, and the order of specific activity was found to be GluV8>>GluScp>GluSW>GluSE. These GluV8 family proteases may be associated with the survival and spreading of bacteria *in vivo* by cleavage of proteinous molecules involved in host defense. GluV8 degrades α_1-protease inhibitor, which is the major inhibitor of elastase. Inactivation of α_1-protease inhibitor then causes activation of elastase released from activated neutrophilic granulocytes, resulting in damage to host tissues (Arvidson, 2006).

In a comparison of amino acid sequence and proteolytic activity, the following essential amino acid residues in the GluV8-protease family were determined. Val_1 is required to exert proper maturation mediated by cleavage between the Xaa-Val bond and for proteolytic activity itself, with Trp_{185}, Val_{188} and Pro_{189} also involved in proteolytic activity (Fig. 9) (Nemoto et al., 2009). The K_m value of native GluSE harboring a combination of $Tyr_{185}Val_{188}Asp_{189}$ was larger than that of GluV8 with $Trp_{185}Val_{188}Pro_{189}$. Amino acid substitutions in these three residues decreased K_m with a constant k_{cat} value (Table 5). These residues can be involved in substrate affinity, which implicates the mechanism of alteration in proteolytic activity among the members of this family.

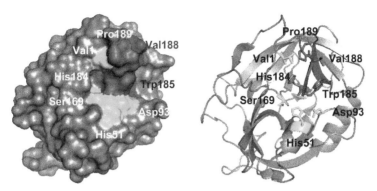

Fig. 9. Amino acid residues involved in proteolytic activity of GluV8 are shown in a three-dimensional structure. The catalytic triad and Val_1 are shown in green, and His_{184} to Pro_{189} and Glu_{191} to Phe_{198}, which form an anti-parallel β-sheet, are shown in red and blue, respectively

Protease	K_m (mM)	k_{cat} (s^{-1})
GluV8 ($W_{185}V_{188}P_{189}$)	0.30±0.08	6147±1117
GluSE ($W_{185}V_{188}P_{189}$)	0.35±0.13	7695±1200
GluSE ($W_{185}V_{188}D_{189}$)	2.84±1.49	8863±1765
GluSE ($Y_{185}V_{188}P_{189}$)	4.15±1.58	7681±3069
GluSE ($W_{185}A_{188}P_{189}$)	1.32±0.10	9059±4205

Table 5. Kinetic parameters of recombinant GluV8 and GluSE with amino acid substitutions at positions 185, 188, and 189

Recently, Iwase et al. (2010) reported that biofilm formation by *S. aureus* was inhibited by GluSE, which also destroyed pre-existing *S. aureus* biofilms. Accordingly, GluSE enhanced the susceptibility of *S. aureus* colonizing the nasal cavity to host immune system components. These observations suggest the existence of bacterial interference among *Staphylococcus* species mediated by GluV8-family proteases in normal microflora. At present, the molecular mechanism remains unclear. It is not easy to speculate how bacterial proteases harbouring the same substrate specificity degrade opponent factors without affecting the corresponding self-factors. Therefore, investigations on the production regulation of GluV8-family proteases and their target molecules are important. Production of GluV8 together with other virulence factors, such as hemolysins and toxins, is regulated by the well-studied system of the accessory gene regulator (*arg*) locus (Ji et al., 1997; Novick 2003). Recent reports have raised the possibility that the *arg* system as well as GluV8 or other extracellular proteases is involved in biofilm detachment (Yarwood et al., 2004; Boles & Horswill, 2008; Martí et al., 2010). Thus, regulation of the biosynthesis of proteinous factors, especially GluV8-family proteases in *Staphylococcus* species, and their relationship with bacterial interference must be elucidated to better understand the molecular mechanism of onset of staphylococcal IE.

5. Acknowledgments

This research was supported by grants-in-aid for scientific research from the Ministry of Education, Science, Sports, and Culture of Japan.

6. References

Aas, J. A., Paster, B. J., Stokes, L. N., Olsen, I. & Dewhirst, F. E. (2005) Defining the normal bacterial flora of the oral cavity. *J. Clin. Microbiol.* vol. 43, pp. 5721-5732, 0095-1137

Alshammary, A., Hervas-Malo, M. & Robinson, J. L. (2008) Pediatric infective endocarditis: Has *Staphylococcus aureus* overtaken viridans group streptococci as the predominant etiological agent? *Can. J. Infect. Des. Med. Microbiol.* vol. 19, pp. 63-68, 1712-9532

Arvidson, S. (2006) Extracellular enzymes, *In: Gram-positive pathogens* (2nd ed.), Eds. Fischetti, V. A., Novick, R. P., Ferretti, J. J., Portnoy, D. A. & Rood, J. I., pp. 478-485, ASM Press, 1-55581-343-7, Washington, D.C.

Berlin, J.A., Abrutyn, E., Strom, B.L., Kinman, J.L., Levison, M.E., Korzeniowski, O.M., Feldman, R.S., Kaye, D. (1995) Incidence of infective endocarditis in the Delaware Valley, 1988-1990. *Am. J. Cardiol.* vol. 76, pp. 933-936, 0002-9149

Boles, B. R. & Horswill, A. R. (2008) *agr*-Mediated dispersal of *Staphylococcus aureus* biofilms. *PLoS Pathog.* vol. 4, e1000052, 1553-7366

Boles, B. R., Thoendel, M., Roth, A. J. & Horswill, A. R. (2010) Identification of genes involved in polysaccharide-independent *Staphylococcus aureus* biofilm formation. *PLoS One* vol. 5, e10146, 1932-6203

Bouvet, A. (1995) Human endocarditis due to nutritionally variant streptococci: *Streptococcus adjacens* and *Streptococcus defectivus. Eur. Heart J.* vol. 16, Suppl B, pp. 24-27, 0195-668x

Carmona, I. T., Dios, P. D., Posse, J. L., Quintela, A. G., Vázquez, C. M. & Iglesias A. C. (2002) An update on infective endocarditis of dental origin. *J. Dent.* vol. 30, 37-40, 0300-5712

Cecchi, E., Forno, D., Imazio, M., Migliardi, A., Gnavi, R., Dal Conte, I., Trinchero, R.; Piemonte Infective Endocarditis Study Group. (2004) New trends in the epidemiological and clinical features of infective endocarditis: results of a multicenter prospective study. *Ital. Heart J.* vol. 5, pp. 249-256, 1129-4728

Collins, M. D. & Lawson, P. A. (2000) The genus *Abiotrophia* (Kawamura *et al.*) is not monophyletic: proposal of *Granulicatella* gen. nov., *Granulicatella adiacens* comb. nov. and *Granulicatella balaenopterae* comb. nov. *Int. J. Syst. Evol. Microbiol.* vol. 50, pp. 365-369, 1466-5026

Coulter, S. N., Schwan, W. R., Ng, E. Y. W., Langhorne, M. H., Ritchie, H. D., Westbrock-Wadman, S., Hutnagle, W. O., Folger, K. R., Bayer, A. S. & Stover, C. K. (1998) *Staphylococcus aureus* genetic loci impacting growth and survival in multiple infection environment. *Mol. Microbiol.* vol. 30, pp.393-404, 0950-382x

Cramton, S. E., Gerke, C., Schnell, N. F., Nichols, W. W. & Götz, F. (1999) The intercellular adhesion (*ica*) locus is present in *Staphylococcus aureus* and is required for biofilm formation. *Infect. Immun.* vol. 67, pp. 5427-5433, 0019-9567

Cucarella, C., Solano, C., Valle, J., Amorena, B., Lasa, Í. & Penadés, J. R. (2001) Bap, a *Staphylococcus aureus* surface protein involved in biofilm formation. *J. Bacteriol.* vol. 183, pp. 2888–2896, 0021-9193

Di Filippo, S., Delahaye, F., Semiond, B., Celard, M., Henaine, R., Ninet, J., Sassolas, F. & Bozio, A. (2006) Current patterns of infective endocarditis in congenital heart disease. *Heart* vol. 92, pp. 1490-1495, 1355-6037

Drapeau, G. R., Boily, Y. & Houmard, J. (1972) Purification and properties of an extracellular protease of *Staphylococcus aureus*. *J. Biol. Chem.* vol. 247, pp. 6720-6726, 0021-9258

Dubin, G., Chmiel, D., Mak, P., Rakwalska, M., Rzychon, M. & Dubin, A. (2001) Molecular cloning and biochemical characterisation of proteases from *Staphylococcus epidermidis*. *Biol. Chem.* vol. 382, pp. 1575-1582, 1431-6730

El-Solh, A. A., Pletrantoni, C., Bhat A., Okada, M., Zambon, J., Aquilina, A. & Berbary, E. (2004) Colonization of dental plaques: A reservoir of respiratory pathogens for hospital-acquired pneumonia in institutionalized elders. *Chest* vol. 126, pp. 1575-1582, 0012-3692

Etienne, J., Fleurette, J., Ninet, J. F., Favet, P. & Gruer, L. D. (1986) Staphylococcal endocarditis after dental extraction. *Lancet* vol. 2, pp. 511-512, 0140-6736

Fedeli, U., Schievano, E., Buonfrate, D., Pellizzer, G. & Spolaore, P. (2011) Increasing incidence and mortality of infective endocarditis: a population-based study through a record-linkage system. *BMI Infect. Dis.* vol. 11:48, doi:10.1186/1471-2334-11-48

Ferreiros, E., Nacinovich, F., Casabé, J. H., Modenesi, J. C., Swieszkowski, S., Cortes, C., Hernan, C. A., Kazelian, L. &Varini, S.; Eira-2 Investigators. (2006) Epidemiologic, clinical, and microbiologic profile of infective endocarditis in Argentina: a national survey. *Am. Heart J.* vol. 151, pp. 545-552, 0002-8703

Frank, K. L. & Patel, R. (2007) Poly-*N*-acetylglucosamine is not a major component of the extacellular matrix in biofilms formed by *icaADBC*-positive *Staphylococcus lugdunensis* isolates. *Infect. Immun.* vol. 75, pp. 4728-4742, 0019-9567

Frenkel, A. & Hirsch, W. (1961) Spontaneous development of L forms of streptococci requiring secretions of other bacteria or sulphydryl compounds for normal growth. *Nature* vol. 191, pp. 728-730, 0028-0836

George, R. H. (1974) The isolation of symbiotic streptococci. *J. Med. Microbiol.* vol. 7, pp. 77-83, 0022-2615

Gerke, C., Kraft, A., Süssmuth, R., Schweitzer, O. & Götz, F. (1998) Characterization of the N-acetylglucosaminyltransferase activity involved in the biosynthesis of the *Staphylococcus epidermidis* polysaccharide intercellular adhesin. *J. Biol. Chem.* vol. 273, pp. 18586-18593, 0021-9258

Goldenberger, D., Künzle, A., Vogt, P., Zbinden, R. & Altwegg, M. (1997) Molecular diagnosis of bacterial endocarditis by broad-range PCR amplification and direct sequencing. *J. Clin. Microbiol.* vol. 35, pp. 2733-2739, 0095-1137

Goldenberg, D. L. (1998) Septic arthritis. *Lancet* vol. 351, pp. 197-202, 0140-6736

Götz, F. (2002) *Staphylococcus* and biofilms. *Mol. Microbiol.* vol. 43, pp. 1367-1378, 0950-382x

Gross, M., Cramton, S. E., Götz, F. & Peschel, A. (2001) Key role of teichoic acid net charge in *Staphylococcus aureus* colonization of artificial surfaces. *Infect. Immun.* vol. 69, pp. 3423-3426, 0019-9567

Guidelines for the prevention and treatment of infective endocarditis (JCS 2003) (2003) *Circ. J.* vol. 67, *Suppl. IV* pp. 1039-1082, 1346-9843 (in Japanese)

Heilmann, Schweitzer, O., Gerke, C., Vanittanakom, N., Mack, D. & Götz, F. (1996) Molecular basis of intercellular adhesion in the biofilm-forming *Staphylococcus epidermidis*. *Mol. Microbiol.* vol. 20, pp. 1083-1091, 0950-382x

Hennig, S., Wai, S. N. & Ziebuhr, W. (2007) Spontaneous switch to PIA-independent biofilm formation in an *ica*-positive *Staphylococcus epidermidis* isolate. *Int. J. Med. Microbiol.* vol. 297, pp. 117-122, 1438-4221

Hoen, B., Alla, F., Béguinot, I., *et al.* (2002) Changing profile of infective endocarditis: Results of a 1-year survey in France. *JAMA* vol. 288, pp. 75-81, 0098-7484

Hussain, M., Herrmann, M., von Eiff, C., Perdreau-Remington, F. & Peters, G. (1997) A 140-kilodalton extracellular protein is essential for the accumulation of *Staphylococcus epidermidis* strains on surfaces. *Infect. Immun.* vol. 65, pp. 519-524, 0019-9567

Ikeda, Y., Ohara-Nemoto, Y., Kimura, S., Ishibashi, K. & Kaneko, K. (2004) PCR-based identification of *Staphylococcus epidermidis* targeting *gseA* encoding the glutamic-acid- specific protease. *Can. J. Microbiol.* vol. 50, pp. 493-498, 0008-4166

Iwase, T., Uehara, Y., Shinji, H., Tajima, A., Seo, H., Takada, K., Agata, T. & Mizunoe, Y. (2010) *Staphylococcus epidermidis* Esp inhibits *Staphylococcus aureus* biofilm formation and nasal colonization. *Nature* vol. 465, pp. 346-349, 0028-0836

Izano, E. A., Amarante, M. A., Kher, W. B. & Kaplan, J. B. (2008) Differential roles of poly-*N*-acetylglucosamine surface polysaccharide and extracellular DNA in *Staphylococcus aureus* and *Staphylococcus epidermidis* biofilms. *Appl. Environ. Microbiol.* Vol. 74, pp. 470-476, 0099-2240

Jackson, M. S., Bagg, J., Gupta, M. N. & Sturrock, R. D. (1999) Oral carrige of staphylococci in patients with rheumatoid arthritis. *Rheumatology* vol 38, pp. 572-575, 1462-0324

Jacobson, J. J., Patel, B., Asher, G., Woolliscroft, J. O. & Schaberg, D. (1997) Oral staphyloccus in older subjects with rheumatoid arthritis. *J. Am. Geriatr. Soc.* vol. 45, pp. 590-593, 0002-8614

Ji, G., Beavis, R. & Novick, R. P. (1997) Bacterial interference caused by autoinducing peptide variants. *Science* vol. 276, pp. 2027-2030, 0036-8075

Kaandorp, C. J. E., Dinant, H. J., van de Laar, M. A. F. J., Moens, H. J. B., Prins, A. P. A. & Dijkmans, B. A. C. (1997) Incidence and source of native and prosthetic joint infection: a community based prospective survey. *Ann. Rheum. Dis.* vol. 56, 470-475, 0003-4967

Karlsson, A. & Arvidson, S. (2002) Variation in extracellular protease production among clinical isolates of *Staphylococcus aureus* due to different levels of expression of the protease repressor *sarA*. *Infect. Immun.* vol. 70, pp. 4239-4246, 0019-9567

Kawamura, Y., Hou, X. G., Sultana, F., Miura, H. & Ezaki, T. (1995) Determination of 16S rRNA sequences of *Streptococcus mitis* and *Streptococcus gordonii* and phylogenetic relationships among members of the genus *Streptococcus*. *Int. J. Syst. Bacteriol.* vol. 45, pp. 406-408, 0020-7713

Kimura, S. & Ohara-Nemoto, Y. (2007) Early childhood caries and childhood periodontal diseases. In: *Pediatric Infectious Diseases Revisited,* Schroten, H. & Wirth, S. (eds), pp. 177-197, Birkhäuser Verlag, Basel, 3-7643-8099-3

Kishi, M., Ohara-Nemoto, Y., Takahashi, M., Kishi, K., Kimura, S. & Yonemitsu, M. (2010) Relationship between oral status and prevalence of periodontopathic bacteria on the tongues of elderly individuals. *J. Med. Microbiol.* vol. 59, pp. 1354-1359, 0022-2615

Koren, O., Spor, A., Felin, J., Fåk, F., Stombaugh, J., Tremaroli, V., Behre, C. J., Knight, R., Fagerberg, B., Ley, R. E. & Bäckhed, F. (2011) Human oral, gut, and plaque microbiota in patients with atherosclerosis. *Proc. Nat. Acad. Sci. USA* vol. 108, pp. 4592-4598, 0027-8424

Mack, D., Fischer, W., Krokotsch, A., Leopold, K., Hartmann, R., Egge, H. & Laufs, R. (1996) The intercellular adhesin involved in biofilm accumulation of *Staphylococcus epidermidis* is a linear β-1,6-linked glucosaminoglycan: purification and structural analysis. *J. Bacteriol.* vol. 178, pp. 175-183, 0021-9193

Maderazo, E. G., Judson, S. & Pasternak, H. (1988) Late infections of total joint prostheses: a review and recommendation for prevention. *Clin. Orthop. Relat. Res.* vol. 229, pp. 131-142, 0009-921x

Marsh, P. D. & Martin, M. V. (2009) *Oral Microbiology* (5th ed.), Churchill Livingstone Elsevier, 978-0-443-10144-1, London

Martí, M., Trotonda, M. P., Tormo-Más, M. Á., Vergara-Irigaray, M., Cheung, A. L., Lasa, I. & Penadés, J. R. (2010) Extracellular proteases inhibit protein-dependent biofilm formation in *Staphylococcus aureus*. *Microbes. Infect.* vol. 12, pp. 55-64, 1286-4579

Moon, J. L., Banbula, A., Oleksy, A., Mayo, J. A. & Travis, J. (2001) Isolation and characterization of a highly specific serine endopeptidase from an oral strain of *Staphylococcus epidermidis*. *Biol. Chem.* vol. 382, pp. 1095-1099, 1431-6730

Murdoch, F. E., Sammons, R. L. & Chapple, I. L. (2004) Isolation and characterization of subgingival staphylococci from periodontitis patients and controls. *Oral Dis.* vol. 10, pp. 155-162, 1354-523X

Murdoch, D.R., Corey, G. R., Hoen, B., et al. (2009) Clinical presentation, etiology, and outcome of infective endocarditis in the 21st century: the International Collaboration on Endocarditis-Prospective Cohort Study. *Arch. Intern. Med.* vol. 169, pp. 463-473, 0003-9926

Nakatani, S., Misutake, K., Hozumi, T., et al. (2003) Current characteristics of infective endocarditis in Japan. An analysis of 848 cases in 2000 and 2001. *Circ. J.* vol. 67, pp. 901-905, 1346-9843

Nemoto, T. K., Ohara-Nemoto, Y., Ono, Y., Kobayakawa, T., Shimoyama, Y., Kimura, S. & Takagi, T. (2008) Characterization of the glutamyl endopeptidase from *Staphylococcus aureus* expressed in *Escherichia coli*. *FEBS J.* vol. 275, pp. 573-587, 1742-464x

Nemoto, T. K., Ono, T., Shimoyama, Y., Kimura, S. & Ohara-Nemoto, Y. (2009) Determination of three amino acids causing alteration of proteolytic activities of staphylococcal glutamyl endopeptidases. *Biol. Chem.* vol. 390, pp. 277-285, 1431-6730

Niwa, K., Nakazawa, M., Tateno, S., Yoshinaga, M. & Terai, M. (2005) Infective endocarditis in congenital heart disease: Japanese national collaboration study. *Heart* vol. 91, pp. 795-800, 1355-6037

Novick, R. P. (2003) Autoinduction and signal transduction in the regulation of staphylococcal virulence. *Mol. Microbiol.* vol. 48, pp. 1429-1449, 0950-382x

Ohara-Nemoto, Y., Tajika, S., Sasaki, M. & Kaneko, M. (1997) Identification of *Abiotrophia adiacens* and *Abiotrophia defectiva* by 16S rRNA gene PCR and restriction fragment length polymorphism analysis. *J. Clin. Microbiol.* vol. 35, pp. 2458-2463, 0095-1137

Ohara-Nemoto, Y., Ikeda, Y., Kobayashi, M., Sasaki, M., Tajika, S. & Kimura, S. (2002) Characterization and molecular coloning of a glutamyl endopeptidases from *Staphylococcus epidermidis*. *Microb. Pathog.* vol. 33, pp. 33-41, 0882-4010

Ohara-Nemoto, Y., Kishi, K., Satho, M., Tajika, S., Sasaki, M., Namioka, A. & Kimura, S. (2005) Infective endocarditis caused by *Granulicatella elegans* originating in the oral cavity. *J. Clin. Microbiol.* vol. 43, pp. 1405-1407, 0095-1137

Ohara-Nemoto, Y., Haraga, H., Kimura, S. & Nemoto, T. K. (2008a) Occurrence of staphylococci in the oral cavities of healthy adults and nasal-oral trafficking of the bacteria. *J. Med. Microbiol.* vol. 57, pp. 95-99, 0022-2615

Ohara-Nemoto, Y., Ono, T., Shimoyama, Y., Kimura, S. & Nemoto, T. K. (2008b) Homologous and heterologous expression and maturation processing of extracellular glutamyl endopeptidases of *Staphylococcus epidermidis*. *Biol. Chem.* vol. 389, pp. 1209-1217, 1431-6730

Okell, C. C., Okell, C. C. & Elliott, S.D. (1935) Bacteriaemia and oral sepsis with special reference to the etiology of subacute endocarditis. *Lancet* vol. 2, pp. 869-872, 0140-6736

Ono, T., Ohara-Nemoto, Y., Shimoyama, Y., Okawara, H., Kobayakawa, T., Baba, T.T., Kimura, S. & Nemoto, T. K. (2010) Amino acid residues modulating the activities of staphylococcal glutamyl endopeptidases. *Biol. Chem.* vol. 391, pp. 1221-1232, 1431-6730

Otto, M. (2009) *Staphylococcus epidermidis* – the 'accidental' pathogen. *Nature Rev. Microbiol.* vol. 7, 555-567, 1740-1526

Percival, R. S., Challacombe, S. J. & Marsh, P. D. (1991) Age-related microbiological changes in the salivary and plaque microflora of healthy adults. *J. Med. Microbiol.* vol. 35, pp. 5-11, 0022-2615

Pompei, R., Caredda, E., Piras, V., Serra, C. & Pintus, L. (1990) Production of bacteriolytic activity in the oral cavity by nutritionally variant streptococci. *J. Clin. Microbiol.* vol. 28, pp. 1623-1627, 0095-1137

Qin, Z., Ou, Y., Yang, L., Zhu, Y., Tolker-Nielsen, T., Molin, S. & Qu, D. (2007) Role of autolysin-mediated DNA release in biofilm formation of *Staphylococcus epidermidis*. *Microbiology* vol. 153, pp. 2083–2092, 1350-0872

Rice, K. C., Mann, E. E., Endres, J. L., Weiss, E. C., Cassat, J. E., Smeltzer, M. S. & Bayles, K. W. (2007) The *cidA* murein hydrolase regulator contributes to DNA release and biofilm development in *Staphylococcus aureus*. *Proc. Natl. Acad. Sci. USA* vol. 104, pp. 8113-8118, 0027-8424

Roggenkamp, A., Abele-Horn, M., Trebesius, K.-H., Tretter, U., Autenrieth, I. B. & Heesemann, J. (1998) *Abiotrophia elegans* sp. nov., a possible pathogen in patients with culture-negative endocarditis. *J. Clin. Microbiol.* vol. 36, pp. 100–104, 0095-1137

Rohde, H., Burandt, E. C., Siemssen, N., Frommelt, L., Burdelski, C., Wurster, S., Scherpe, S., Davies, A. P., Harris, L. G., Horstkotte, M. A., Knobloch, J. K., Ragunath, C.,

Kaplan, J. B. & Mack, D. (2007) Polysaccharide intercellular adhesin or protein factors in biofilm accumulation of *Staphylococcus epidermidis* and *Staphylococcus aureus* isolated from prosthetic hip and knee joint infections. *Biomaterials* vol. 28, pp. 1711-1720, 0142-9612

Ruoff, K. L. (1991) Nutritionally variant streptococci. *Clin. Microbiol. Rev.* vol. 4, pp. 184-190, 0893-8512

Ruoff, K. L. (2007) *Aerococcus, Abiotrophia*, and other aerobic catalase-negative, gram-positive cocci. *In Manual of Clinical Microbiology*, (9th ed.) Eds. Murray, P. R. *et al.* ASM Press, pp. 443-454, 1-55581-371-2, Washington, D.C.

Ryan, M. J., Kavanagh, R., Wall, P. G. & Hazleman, B. L. (1997) Bacterial joint infections in England and Wales: analysis of bacterial isolates over a four year period. *Br. J. Rheumatol.* vol 36, pp. 370-373, 0263-7103

Sadovskaya, I., Vinogradov, E., Flahaut, S., Kogan, G. & Jabbouri, S. (2005) Extracellular carbohydrate-containing polymers of a model biofilm-producing strain, *Staphylococcus epidermidis* RP62A. *Infect. Immun.* vol. 73, pp. 3007–3017, 0019-9567

Sandre, R. M. & Shafran, S. D. (1996) Infective endocarditis: review of 135 cases over 9 years. *Clin. Infect. Dis.* vol. 22, pp. 276-286, 1058-4838

Sasaki, M., Ohara-Nemoto, Y., Tajika, S., Kobayashi, M., Ikeda, Y., Kaneko, M. & Takagi, T. (1998) Purification and characterization of glutamic acid-specific protease from *Staphylococcus epidermidis. Jpn. J. Oral Biol.* vol. 40, pp. 542-548, 0385-0137

Sato, S., Kanamoto, T. & Inoue, M. (1999) *Abiotrophia elegans* strains comprise 8% of the nutritionally variant streptococci isolated from the human mouse. *J. Clin. Microbiol.* vol. 37, pp. 2553-2556, 0095-1137

Shimoyama, Y., Sasaki, M., Ohara-Nemoto, Y., Nemoto, T. K., Ishikawa, T. & Kimura, S. (in press) Rapid identification of *Abiotrophia/Granulicatella* species using by 16S rRNA PCR and RFLP. *Interface Oral Health Science 2010*

Smith, A. J., Jackson, M. S. & Bagg, J. (2001) The ecology of *Staphylococcus* species in the oral cavity. *J. Med. Microbiol.* vol. 50, pp. 940-946, 0022-2615

Strom, B. L., Abrutyn, E., Berlin, J. A., Kinman, J. L., Feldman, R. S., Stolley, P. D., Levison, M. E., Korzeniowski, O. M. & Kaye, D. (1998) Dental and cardiac risk factors for infective endocarditis: a population-based case-control study. *Ann. Intern. Med.* vol. 129, pp. 761–769, 0003-4819

Strom, B. L., Abrutyn, E., Berlin, J. A., Kinman, J. L., Feldman, R. S., Stolley, P. D., Levison, M. E., Korzeniowski, O. M. & Kaye, D. (2000) Risk factors for infective endocarditis. Oral hygiene and nondental exposures. *Circulation* vol. 102, pp. 2842-2848, 0009-7322

Tleyjeh, I. M., Steckelberg, J. M., Murad, H. S., Anavekar, N. S., Ghomrawi, H. M., Mirzoyev, Z., Houstafa, S. E., Hoskin, T. L., Mandrekar, J. N., Wilson, W. R. & Baddour, L. M. (2005) Temporal trends in infective endocarditis. A population-based study in Olmsted County, Minnesota. *JAMA* vol. 293, pp. 3022-3028, 0098-7484

Tuohy, M. J., Procop, G. W. & Washington, J. A. (2000) Antimicrobial susceptibility of *Abiotrophia adiacens* and *Abiotrophia defectiva. Diagn. Microbiol. Infect. Dis.* vol. 38, pp. 189-191, 0732-8893

Vinogradov, E., Sadovskaya, I., Li, J. & Jabbouri, S. (2006) Structural elucidation of the extracellular and cell-wall teichoic acids of *Staphylococcus aureus* MN8m, a biofilm forming strain. *Carbohydr. Res.* vol. 341, pp. 738–743, 0008-6215

Yarwood, J. M., Bartels, D. J., Volper, E. M. & Greenberg, E. P. (2004) Qurum sensing in *Staphylococcus aureus* biofilms. *J. Bacteriol.* vol. 186, pp. 1838-1850, 0021-9193

Yoshinaga, M., Niwa, K., Niwa, A., Ishiwada, N., Takahashi, H., Echigo, S., Nakazawa, M., & Japanese Society of Pediatric Cardiology and Cardiac Surgery. (2008) Risk factors for in-hospital mortality during infective endocarditis in patients with congenital heart disease. *Am. J. Cardiol.* vol. 101, pp. 114-118, 0002-9149

7

Radiology in Infective Endocarditis

C. Prados, C. Carpio, A. Santiago, I. Silva and R. Álvarez-Sala
Pulmonology Service, La Paz University Hospital, Autónoma University, Madrid
Spain

1. Introduction

In the last 50 years, the incidence of infective endocarditis (IE) has remained between 2 and 6 per 100.000 individuals in the general population per year and its mortality has fluctuated between 10% and 30%, depending on the type of pathogen. Historically, chronic rheumatic heart disease had being the primary risk factor for IE but in the last years, new at-risk groups have emerged like individuals undergoing hemodialysis, patients with catheters and elderly people with degenerative valve lesions. IE is characterized by the infection of the endocardium, most commonly by bacteria. Although the primary focus of the infection is confined to the endocardium, microbial shedding by continuous bacteremia and embolization of vegetation fragments makes IE a true systemic infection. This disease, therefore, is positioned at the crossroads of multiple medical specialties, including cardiology, cardiac surgery, infectious diseases, internal medicine, neurology, and intensive care. Valve vegetations are specific pathologic findings of this disease. They are the result of the combination of thrombus with bacteria and leucocytes. The size and mobility of valvular vegetations are important predictors of whether or not the patient will develop septic emboli. These lesions usually affect valve endocardium, but it also could involve papillary muscles, mural endocardium and the great vessels. IE is fatal if it is not treated early with antibiotics. Negative prognostic factors are fungal etiology, involvement of the aortic valve, and presence of large vegetations. Patients with a left-sided endocarditis have a higher mortality in comparison to patients with right-sided endocarditis

The mean age of patients with IE has increased from 30 years in the 1950s, to 50 years in the 1980s. The higher frequency of IE diagnosis in older individuals probably reflects the clustering of more than one risk factor in the elderly. The results of epidemiological studies vary depending on the population analyzed and the microbial pathogens tend to differ between the various groups.

2. Classification

IE can be classified in four categories:

- Native valve endocarditis
- Intravenous drug abuse endocarditis (IVDA)
- Prosthetic valve endocarditis
- Pacemaker endocarditis and nosocomial endocarditis

Left-sided native valve endocarditis is the most frequent form of endocarditis, representing more than 60% of all cases. In-hospital mortality is approximately 15%. Pre-existing lesions can favor attachment of circulating bacteria and promote IE. Frequently, congenital or acquired valve diseases are present (rheumatic fever, degenerative cardiopathies, mitral valve prolapse). Mitral –valve prolapsed is a relatively common condition and have a 10–100-fold increased risk of IE. Degenerative valve lesions are present in up to 25% of patients with IE and they involve local inflammation, microulcers, and microthrombi of the endothelium. Degenerative valve lesions might increase the risk of IE in up to 50% of patients older than 60 years of age. Alpha-hemolytic streptococci or enterococci typically are the causative agents of this type endocarditis.

IVDA endocarditis usually occurs on healthy right heart valves, and 50% of these infections involve the tricuspid valve. Although highly population-specific, right-sided IE has represented up to 5–10% of cases in general surveys. This form of IE has a better prognosis than left-sided IE and in-hospital mortality is <10%, although mortality of up to 50% has been observed in patients with AIDS, especially in advanced cases. Intravenous-drug users, including those with HIV, are a group that primarily consists of relatively young adults. The risk of IE is approximately four to five times higher in those with < 200 CD4 per mm³. The tricuspid valve is usually affected in these patients and Staphylococcus aureus is the most common causative organism.

Prosthetic valve endocarditis is the most-severe form of IE, and is associated with high mortality that ranges from 20% to >40%. It occurs in 1–5% of patients with prosthetic valves and accounts for up to 20% of all cases of IE. It is classified as 'early' or 'late' infection on the basis of the time period between surgery and the onset of IE. Early and late prosthetic valve endocarditis are defined, as occurring either within or more than 12 months after surgery, respectively. Early prosthetic valve endocarditis is often caused by surgery-related and drug-resistant microbes such as methicillin-resistant staphylococci and late endocarditis is due to infection with oral streptococci and Gram-negative bacteria of the HACEK group.

Pacemaker endocarditis are produced by infections of these devices within a few months of implantation. The rate of pacemaker endocartditis is estimated at 0.55 cases per 1,000 pacemakers recipients per year. These infections always require ablation of the material in addition to antibiotic therapy. Of pacemaker infections, 75% are produced by staphylococci.

3. Etiology and pathophysiology

The pathogens involved in IE depend on the different categories of endocarditis. The most frequent IE pathogens are Gram-positive bacteria (S. aureus, Streptococcus spp., and enterococci) and they are responsible for more than 80% of all IE cases. These bacteria have great ability to adhere to and colonize damaged valves and are equipped with several surface adhesins that mediate attachment to extracellular host matrix proteins. The clumping factor A and the fibronectin-binding protein A are involved in valve colonization and invasion of S. aureus. Fibrinogen-binding mediates the primary attachment of the bacteria to nonbacterial thrombotic endocarditis, and subsequent binding of fibronectin triggers endothelial cell internalization, followed by local proinflammatory and procoagulant responses.

Skin microorganisms are responsible for the vast majority of infections in IVDA endocarditis but contamination of drugs and material employed by drug abusers, also contribute to the bacteremia. Aortic and mitral valves are affected in 25% of cases of IVDA endocarditis. The pathogenic mechanisms that explain the increased prevalence of right sided IE in injection drug users are not fully elucidated. Damage to the right sided valves from injected particulate matter in the setting of injected bacterial loads is thought to be important, while subtle abnormalities of immune function may also have a role in pathogenesis. Cocaine use is associated with an increased incidence of endocarditis greater than heroin use, but this finding is not fully explained.

Pulmonary valve is only involved in less than 2% of cases. It is also reported that 6% of patients presents both right and left endocarditis at the same time.

With respect to the pathophysiology, there are many mechanisms proposed to the development of this disease. Endothelial damage can be caused by turbulent blood flow associated with congenital heart disease or prosthetic valves, by electrodes or catheters, or, in intravenous-drug users, from repeated intravenous injection of particulate material. Alternatively, endothelial damage can result from inflammation, for example in patients with rheumatic carditis or in elderly individuals with degenerative valve lesions. Other theories, however, defend the so-called "immunological hypothesis" which explains that the valve affection is secondary to immunological mechanisms that cause local inflammation.

4. Clinical manifestations

Symptoms of IE are related to the infectious condition of the process. General manifestations like persistent fever, chills, pleuritic chest pain, cough and hemoptysis have been described. Embolic events occur in approximately one-third of cases, more frequently in patients with intravenous drug use, right-sided endocarditis or positive blood cultures.

The most common extra-cardiac organ system involved in infective endocarditis is the central nervous system and could produce embolic stroke, intracranial hemorrhage, intracranial mycotic aneurysm, brain abscess and meningitis. With respect to the respiratory system, it has been reported septic pulmonary embolism like a clinical presentation of this condition. In right-sided endocarditis, pulmonary embolic manifestations are frequently present. Septic pulmonary emboli are detected in more than 80% of cases, and may be associated with pleuritic chest pain and dyspnea.

5. Radiology

A chest radiograph should be done routinely but the findings are not specified. Fifty percent of patients with IVDA endocarditis have radiologic opacities and 50-60 % of injection drug users with definite IE have multiple pulmonary opacities (figure 1 and figure 2). The typical radiograph pattern of septic emboli is peripheral, poorly marginated bilateral lung nodules that often demonstrate cavitary changes and moderately thick irregular walls. Also cardiomegaly, pleural effusion and radiographic signs of left heart failure (septal thickening, air bronchogram, pleural effusion) are reported.

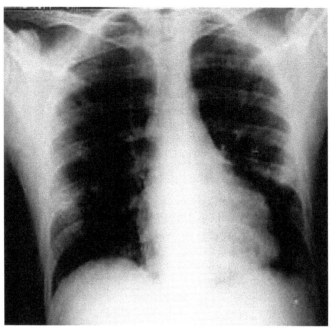

Fig. 1. Chest X-ray showing bilateral opacities and nodules, corresponding to septi emboli

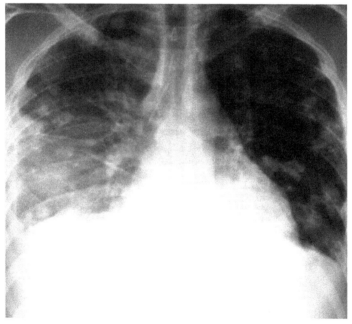

Fig. 2. Chest X-ray showing bilateral opacities. Also it can be observed the presence of pleural fluid

Computed tomography findings include:

- Peripheral triangle opacities, corresponding to regions of pulmonary infarcts produced by septic embolism.
- Peripheral, poorly marginated bilateral lung nodules.
- Cavitary nodules with thick irregular walls. These nodules typically measure 5-35 mm, have a peripheral and basilar predominance, and demonstrate air-bronchograms. The nodule may increase in number and change from day to day (figure 3).
- "Feeding vessel sign" that consists of a distinct vessel leading directly into the center of a nodule.
- Radiologic findings suggestive of empyema like pleural effusion, thickening and enhacement of the visceral and parietal pleurae and inflammation of the extrapleural fat. Also, empyema had been described as a pleural collection that is immnobile on decubitus views. Pleural fluid, pericardic fluid and pneumothorax.
- Unilateral or bilateral interstitial lung infiltrate.

In many instances, these radiological findings precede the clinical manifestations of IE. Also, the follow up of septic emboli could be performed by computed tomography.

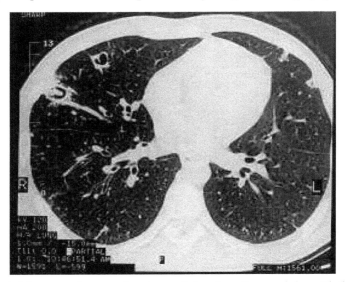

Fig. 3. Computed tomography scan showing peripheral cavitary nodules with thick irregular walls from 1 to 3 cm of size

These radiological findings are more common in IVDA endocarditis but also they can be found, less commonly, in other types of right IE, like endocarditis associated to pacemaker and intravascular devices. It is important to differentiate other radiologic presentation of IVDA, like ground-glass opacities, pulmonary hemorrhage, air trapping and pulmonary hypertension. When IE affects left chambers, radiographic findings are less frequent. Furthermore, they only appear in the context of heart complications: increased cardiothoracic ratio (secondary to pericardial effusion) and signs of left heart failure resulting from chordal rupture or valve failure.

6. Conclusion

Although echocardiography is the gold standard in the diagnosis of IE, the presence of many radiological findings could suggest its diagnosis.

7. References

Bittermann V, Pros SA. Manifestaciones osteoarticulares de endocarditis. *Semin Fund Esp Reumatol*. 2010;11:152-8.

Nandakumar R, Raju G. Isolated tricuspid valve endocarditis in nonaddicted patients: A diagnostic challenge. *Am J Med Sci* 1997;314:207-12.

Lacassin F, Leport C. Infectious endocarditis, risk factors, prevention. Research group for infectious endocarditis and jury of the consensus conference. *Rev Med Interne*. 1993; 14(9):871-6.

Clifford SP, Eykyn SJ, Oakley CM. Sthaphylococcal tricuspid valve endocarditis in patients with structurally normal hearts and no evidence of narcotic abuse. *QJM* 1994;87:755-7.

Naidoo DP. Right-sided endocarditis in the non-drug addict. Postgrad Med J 1993;69:615-20.

Prados C, Galera R, Santiago A. Unilateral interstitial lung pattern as a first sign of a bacterial endocarditis. *Arch Bronconeumol*. 2010;46:206-7.

Nguyen E, Silva I, Souza C, Müller N. Pulmonary complications of illicit drug use differential diagnosis based on CT findings. *J Thorac Imaging* 2007;22:199-206.

8

Ocular Complications of Endocarditis

Ozlem Sahin
Middle East Technical University Health Sciences Department of Ophthalmology,
Ankara
Turkey

1. Introduction

Cardiac complications are the most common complications in patients with infective endocarditis, and they can be related to significant mortality and morbidity. (1) Extra-cardiac manifestations along with their historical descriptions such as splinter hemorrhages, emboli, Osler's nodes, Janeway and Bowman lesions of the eye, Roth's spots, patechiae and clubbing generally result from thromboemboli or septic emboli. (2) Inflammatory complications may occur as a result of septic emboli, and these include endogenous (metastatic) endophthalmitis, focal abscess, and vasculitis. (3) In this chapter we mainly focus on the endogenous endophthalmitis arising as a complication of infective endocarditis.

Endogenous (metastatic) endophthalmitis is an inflammatory condition of the intraocular structures including the aqueous, iris, lens, ciliary body, vitreous, choroid and retina. (4-6) It results from the hematogenous spread of organisms from a distant source of infection, most commonly infective endocarditis, gastrointestinal tract and urinary tract infections and wound infections. (7-9) Other sources of infection have included pharyngitis, pneumonia, septic arthritis and meningitis. (10,11) Compared with endophthalmitis following trauma or surgery, endogenous endophthalmitis is relatively rare, accounting 2-8% of all reported endophthalmitis cases. (5) However, endogenous endophthalmitis carries with it the danger of bilateral infection in 15-25% of cases. (6,12)

2. Epidemiology

Endogenous endophthalmitis has been reported to occur at any age and no sexual predilection. (13) However, in the recent years the mean age of endogenous endophthalmitis has shifted to 65 years possibly because of the reduction in the incidence of rheumatic heart disease. (14)

The mean incidence of endogenous endophthalmitis was reported as1.8 cases/year, and 48.1% of patients presented were seen as outpatients. (15) Endogenous bacterial endophthalmitis is recognized as a major cause of visual loss with an associated high mortality rate. (16,17) It is considered a diagnostic challenge in the early stages of the disease, with 16% to 63% of cases being initially misdiagnosed (18). In unilateral cases, the right eye is twice as likely to become infected as the left eye, probably because of the more proximal location and direct blood flow to the right carotid artery. (19)

3. Classification of endogenous endophthalmitis

A classification system introduced by Greenwald et al. takes into consideration the affected areas of the globe and the associated visual prognosis. (20) It is divided as focal anterior or posterior, diffuse anterior or posterior and panophthalmitis. (20) Anterior focal endophthalmitis manifests as localized inflammatory nodules or plaques in the iris and/or ciliary body associated with iridocyclitis and minimal hypopyon. (5,21) (Fig. 1) Intraocular pressure varies from normal to high. (5,21) The anterior vitreous has no or minimal inflammation. (5,21) The retina is normal. (5,21) The prognosis in these cases is good. (21) Anterior diffuse endophthalmitis is characterized by a more severe anterior segment inflammation associated with conjunctival chemosis, marked anterior chamber reaction with fibrin clots and significant hypopyon that hampers the view of retina. (5,21) (Fig. 2)

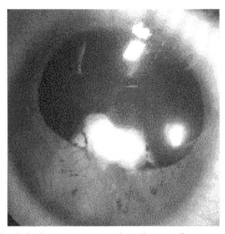

Fig. 1. Anterior focal endophthalmitis presented with an inflammatory nodule in the iris extending from the ciliary body

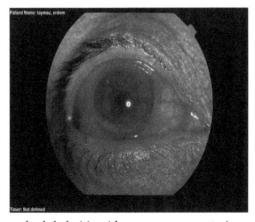

Fig. 2. Anterior diffuse endophthalmitis with a more severe anterior segment inflammation associated with conjunctival chemosis, marked anterior chamber reaction with fibrin clots and significant hypopyon

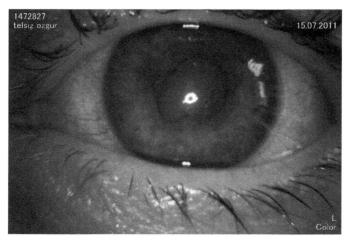

Fig. 3. Anterior diffuse endophthalmitis with posterior synechia and corneal haze

Intraocular pressure is typically elevated. (22) Corneal opacification may occur. (22) (Fig. 3) It is an ocular emergency and if not promptly and adequately treated the infection can spread to the entire eye. (22) The visual prognosis is excellent with aggressive and appropriate treatment. Blindness usually results from delay in treatment. (22) Posterior focal endophthalmitis manifests as white-yellowish retinal or choroidal lesions associated with retinal hemorrhages and vitreous cells and/or debris. (23) (Fig. 4) Infections caused by Gram-positive organisms may show multifocal lesions. (23) However, Gram-negative infections usually cause a single large choroidal abscess involving the posterior pole. (24,25) (Fig. 5) The anterior chamber reaction is usually mild with or without keratic precipitates. (23) (Fig. 6) The intraocular pressure varies from low to normal. (23) Posterior diffuse endophthalmitis may present as multiple whitish lesions located inside the vessels or in the

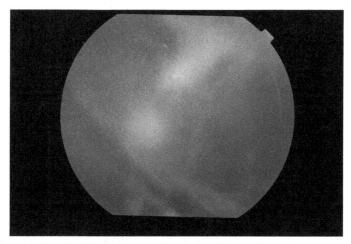

Fig. 4. Posterior focal endophthalmitis manifested as white-yellowish retinal or choroidal lesions associated with vitreous cells and/or debris

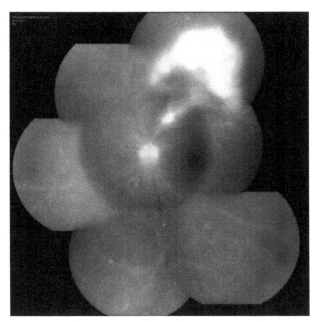

Fig. 5. A single large choroidal abscess involving the posterior pole

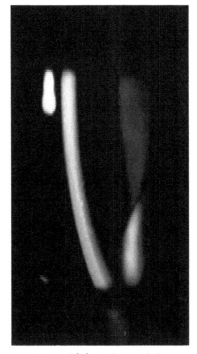

Fig. 6. Mild anterior chamber reaction with keratic precipitates

retina with perivascular hemorrhages in the early stages of the disease. (26) As the infection progresses, the retina becomes necrotic, and vitreous abscess frequently occur. (26) (Fig. 7) The anterior segment is also involved with forward spread of the infection and hypopyon is formed as the disease progresses. (26) (Fig. 8) The intraocular pressure is low. (26) The poor visual prognosis is most likely due to retinal ischemia as a result of occlusion of central retinal artery by a septic embolus. (26) Panophthalmitis is inflammation of all coats of the eye including intraocular structures. (27-29) It presents with marked lid edema, proptosis and limitation of ocular movements. (28) (Fig. 9) All details of anterior as well as posterior chamber are lost because of the prominent hypopyon. (29) (Fig. 10) Typically the intraocular pressure is high. (29)It is a disastrous and rapidly developing infection that destroys the globe and invades the orbit, resulting in blindness, phthisis or enucleation. (28,29) Depending of the virulence of pathogen, progression of panophthalmitis may be life threatening. (28)

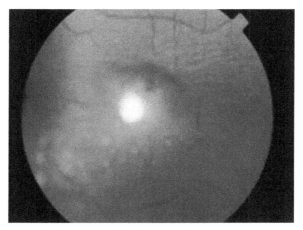

Fig. 7. Necrotic / hemorrhagic retina with vitreous abscess

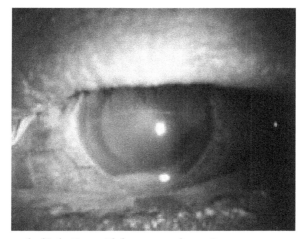

Fig. 8. Forward spread of infection with hypopyon formation

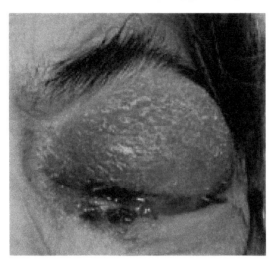

Fig. 9. Panophthalmitis with marked lid edema and proptosis

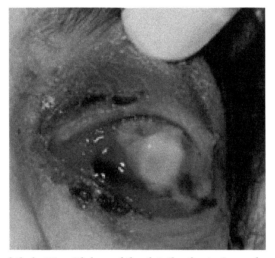

Fig. 10. Severe panophthalmitis with loss of the details of anterior and posterior segments of the eye

4. Pathogenesis

In endogenous endophthalmitis the microorganisms enter into the uveal tract or retinal circulation as scattered organisms or in a bolus, and lodge in small capillaries. (30,31) To invade ocular tissues and produce infection the organisms must cross the blood-ocular barrier either by direct invasion (septic emboli) or by changes in vascular endothelium caused by substrates released during infection. (30) They establish a septic focus that can develop in the retina prior to breaking into the vitreous. (30) The infectious embolus is usually in proximity to the retinal vessels. (30) If a large septic embolus pass through the central retinal artery and disseminates throughout the retina, retinal necrosis and ischemia may occur. (30) This allows the microorganisms to quickly invade the vitreous and further the anterior segment, causing inflammation of intraocular tissues (panuveitis) that may be mixed-up a non-infectious inflammatory disease. (31) Similarly, in cases of fungal endophthalmitis a localized inflammatory reaction surrounding a small nidus of fungi forms in the inner choroid, breaks through Bruch's membrane into the retina forming a microabscess and spreads into the vitreous cavity. (31) It is a destructive process that has a poor visual prognosis that the visual loss rate reaches up to 37.5%. (30) The final visual outcome in patients with endogenous bacterial endophthalmitis in the recent 12 years has not differed significantly from five decades ago. (31) Under normal circumstances, the blood-ocular barrier provides a natural resistance against invading organisms. (30) Destruction of intraocular tissues may be due to direct invasion of the organism and/or from inflammatory mediators of the immune system. (30,31) In any type of endophthalmitis, bacteria are introduced into the intraocular environment, encountering a site of immunological inactivity. (30) The intraocular environment is termed an "immune privileged site", devoid of inflammatory mediators and cells present that would otherwise fight infection. (32) The blood-ocular barrier facilitates maintenance of a sterile environment in the interior of the eye contributing to the immune privileged site. (32) In this environment initial immune responses that would typically handle infection are delayed or absent, providing an optimum growth medium for the organisms that reach the area. (32) Eventually, organisms are recognized and inflammation initiates in an effort to handle the infection. (30) The extent of inflammation in the eye is during endophthalmitis has been shown to be organism dependent. (30,31) The course of endophthalmitis, treatment effectiveness and visual outcome can be unpredictable. (33) Clinical presentation of the disease depends, in part, on the relative virulence of the infecting pathogen, the mechanism of introduction into the eye and how quickly treatment is initiated. (33) Other factors that affect the outcome of infection include the patients' age, how vulnerable the infecting agent is to antibiotic therapy and the anatomic condition of the eye during infection. (33) Clinical studies have reported that increased time between infection and treatment is associated with a worse visual outcome. (19,34) Endophthalmitis may be as subtle as white nodules on the lens capsule, iris, retina, or choroid. (35) It can also be as ubiquitous as inflammation of all the ocular tissues, leading to a globe full of purulent exudate. (36) In addition, inflammation can spread to involve the orbital soft tissue. (37)

5. Mortality/morbidity

Decreased vision and permanent loss of vision are common complications of endophthalmitis. (33,34) Patients may require enucleation to eradicate a blind and painful eye. (38) Mortality is related to the patient's comorbidities and the underlying medical problem, especially when considering the etiology of hematogenous spread in endogenous infections. (39,40)

6. Clinical presentations

Bacterial endophthalmitis usually presents acutely with pain, redness, lid swelling, and decreased visual acuity. (11,16,22) Specific signs have been described which may suggest a specific infecting organism. For example, Bacillus infections characteristically demonstrate chocolate brown anterior chamber exudates with a ring-shaped white corneal infiltrate. (41) Serratia infections may be associated with a pink or dark hypopyon. (42,43) An eye with Klebsiella or Group B Streptoccoccus endogenous endophthalmitis often has a pupillary hypopyon. (44,45) The hypopyon associated with Group B Streptococcus often does not organize and shifts to occupy the most dependent portion of the anterior chamber. This has been termed a "sliding hypopyon". (46) Fungal endophthalmitis may present with an indolent course over days to weeks. (47) Symptoms are often blurred vision, pain and decreased visual acuity. (47) Individuals with candidal infection may present with high fever, followed several days later by ocular symptoms. (48) Persistent fever of unknown origin may be associated with an occult retinochoroidal fungal infiltrate. (48) A characteristic sign of endogenous Candida endophthalmitis is a creamy, white, well-circumscribed lesion, involving the retina and choroid in the posterior pole. (48) Aspergillus endogenous endophthalmitis, although less common, is frequently a more fulminant disease. (40) Nearly all patients have anterior chamber cells and keratic precipitates. (40) The inflammation may result in hypopyon, pupillary membrane, rubeosis iridis, and an anterior chamber inflammatory mass. (40) Posteriorly, chorioretinitis may appear as fluffy yellow-white elevated chorioretinal opacities. (49) Gravitational layering of the inflammatory cells may produce a subhyaloid or subretinal "hypopyon" especially since subretinal and subretinal pigment epithelial infection tends to occur with Aspergillus. (49) Retinal detachment mat complicate the infection. (40) Retinal haemorrhages and perivasculitis may be present. (40) Ultimately full thickness retinal necrosis may occur. (40) The earlier signs of endogenous endophthalmitis include Roth's spot (round, white retinal spots surrounded by hemorrhage) (Fig. 11), hemorrhagic spots in the conjunctiva, superficial or profound retinal hemorrhage, and retinal periphlebitis. (20-22) The occlusion of small arterioles may produce cotton-wool spots, or if the larger vessels are involved, branch retinal or central retinal artery obstruction. (20-22) Slit-lamp examination reveales ciliary injection, keratic precipitates (KP), mild to moderate cells and flare in the anterior chamber or severe iritis with hypopyon formation and fibrin precipitates. (21,22) Ophthalmoscopy shows infiltrations of the retina and vitreous, retinal vasculitis and retinal hemorrhage or dense vitreous opacities progressing to white mass obstructing fundus view. (26,27) If the fundus

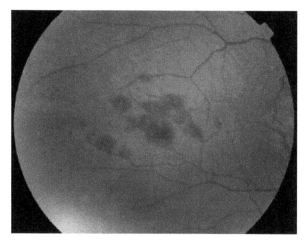

Fig. 11. Roth Spots characterized by round, white retinal spots surrounded by hemorrhage

view is obscured, imaging with optical coherence tomography, ocular ultrasonography, electroretinogram tests are useful in displaying the extent of vitreous involvement, choroidal abscesses, retinal detachment and scleral thickening. (16,18,22) Computed tomography scans allow high resolution orbital imaging in cases of suspected panophthalmitis to detect abscess formation or confirm the presence of contiguous orbital involvement. (37)

7. Causes

Individuals at risk for developing endogenous endophthalmitis usually have comorbidities that predispose them to infection. These include conditions like diabetes mellitus, chronic renal failure, cardiac valvular disorders, prosthetic heart valves, systemic lupus erythematosus, AIDS, leukemia, gastrointestinal malignancies, neutropenia, lymphoma, alcoholic hepatitis, intravenous drug abuse, and bone marrow transplantation. (50,51) Sources of endophthalmitis include most commonly endocarditis followed by urinary tract infection, wound infection and meningitis. (4) Additionally, pharyngitis, pulmonary infection, septic arthritis, pyelonephritis and intraabdominal abscess have also been implicated as sources of infection. (10) About 25% of the cases are bilateral and usually caused by Meningococcus, E.coli and Klebsiella species. (52,53) The most common cause in two-thirds of the infections is Gram-positive bacteria. (31,33) Although the most common agent was S.aureus (25% of patients), the most common group was streptococcus (32%). (31,33) Endogenous endophthalmitis in adults caused by group B Streptococcus has been reported rarely and is almost exclusively related to infective endocarditis. (7,54) Gram-negative organisms cause 32-37% of all endogenous endophthalmitis cases and typically have poor visual outcomes because these infections are difficult to treat. (5,55,56) The low prevalence of Gram-negative bacteria amongst the causative organisms of both infective endocarditis and endogenous endophthalmitis might be related to the absence of an outer capsule, which makes them sensitive to complement mediated lysis and other humoral innate immune defenses, and the lack of surface proteins that specifically bind host matrix molecules and prosthetic material. (57) Moreover, a much higher inoculums of Gram-negative than Gram-positive organisms is required to induce infective endocarditis in laboratory animals. (57) Although aggressive therapy was given, the visual prognosis for all these patients was poor. (56,57) E. coli emphysematous endophthalmitis is a very rare and severe variety of E. coli endophthalmitis. (58,59) The mechanism of emphysematous endophthalmitis has been postulated that a high concentration of glucose in the eye tissue may provide a substrate that bacteria can ferment to produce carbondioxide and hydrogen. (58) A computerized tomography scan of the orbits demonstrate gas bubble in the eye globe indicating emphysematous endophthalmitis. (59) Extra-intestinal pathogenic E.coli (ExPEC) are able to colonize tissue outside the gastrointestinal tract and contain a variety of virulence factors that may enable the pathogens to invade and induce infections in the cardiac endothelia. (57,60) These cases are further complicated by spondylodiscitis and bilateral endophthalmitis. (60) Endogenous endophthalmitis is usually associated with Gram-negative bacteria, most commonly Klebsiella pneumonia (77.4%) among the East Asian population. (6,61,62) The patients at highest risk are diabetic patients with hepatobiliary infections. (6,61) Klebsiella pneumonia endogenous endophthalmitis is a severe but potentially subclinical disease. (62) Early diagnosis requires a high index of suspicion and recognition of risk factors including Asian ancestry and other sources of systemic infection including most commonly liver abscess. (6,61) In contrast, in the Caucasian population, Gram-positive cocci including Staphylococcus aureus, Streptococcus pneumonia and other streptococcal species are the most common causes of bacterial endogenous endophthalmitis. (31,33) Septic metastasis to the iris is a rare manifestation of endogenous endophthalmitis presented with acute painful red eye, hypopyon and iris abscess that might be caused by S.aureus. (63) Subacute bacterial endocarditis caused by viridians streptococci is characterized by a lingering start of the disease with high temperature of unknown origin and an unspecific feeling of illness. (64,65) The ophthalmological findings can manifest itself before the diagnosis of the underlying disease is made. (65) Complications such as blindness after fulminant endophthalmitis and death can be avoided through quick diagnosis and treatment. (64,65) Group B Streptococcus endogenous endophthalmitis is a devastating condition with poor visual prognosis despite therapy. (66,67) It is a rare condition that 17 cases have been reported since 1985. (7) Group B Streptococcus endogenous endophthalmitis was found to arise from hematogenous spread from endocarditis at a rate of 33.3%. (7) Increasing incidence of invasive Group B Streptococcus infection with its varying manifestations including metastatic endophthalmitis has been reported recently in adults with predisposing illnesses. (54,68) Streptococcus anginosus is a member of Streptococcus milleri group and is a commensal found in the mouth, nasopharnyx, throat and sinuses. (69) It is associated with infective endocarditis with a longer than average duration of evolution before diagnosis. (70) S. anginosus should also be considered in the differential diagnosis of a slowly progressive endogenous endophthalmitis when fungal infection is considered likely. (70) Bartonella henselae and Tropheryma whipplei are rare pathogens in humans and were recently recognized as important causative agents of culture-negative endocarditis that the bacteria are indentified by polymerase chain reaction analysis. (71,72) Exposure to cats is an important risk factor for B.henselae which is the causative agent of cat scratch disease characterized by persistent regional lymhadenopathy. (73) B. henselae is responsible for endocarditis in patients with valvular diseases, and may induce retinitis. (73) Whipple's disease is characterized by wide range of clinical manifestations involving diarrhea, weight loss, night sweats, arthritis, vitritis retinitis and papillitis. (74)

Fungal organisms can occur in up to 50% of all cases of endogenous endophthalmitis. (57) Candida albicans is by far the most frequent cause (75-80% of fungal cases). (57) Since 1980, candidal infections reported in intravenous drug users have increased. (57) The number of people at risk may be increasing because of the spread of AIDS, more frequent use of immunosuppressive agents, and more invasive procedures. (57,75) The classic finding of Candida endophthalmitis is white chorioretinal infiltrates with fluffy white vitreous opacities described as "string of pearls" appearance. (76,77) The chorioretinitis may progress and satellite lesions may develop adjacent to the primary lesions. (77) Occasionally anterior uveitis, scleritis and panophthalmitis may also occur. (77) Aspergillus endogenous endophthalmitis, although less common, is frequently a more fulminent disease. (76) It has a predilection for the postequatorial fundus. (78) A confluent yellowish infiltrate is usually seen in the macula beginning in the choroid or subretinal space. (78) Histologically, the retinal and choroidal lesions are angiocentric. (76) Unlike candida endophthalmitis, in which the vitreous is the primary focus of infection, aspergillus endophthalmitis is marked by retinal and choroidal vessel invasion and subretinal pigment epithelial and subretinal infection. (76) The lesions can progress to retinal vascular occlusion and full-thickness retinal necrosis. (78) Intraretinal hemorrhages usually occur. (78) Eventually the infection spreads into the vitreous, producing dense vitritis, and into the anterior segment, producing varying degrees of cell/flare and hypopyon in the anterior chamber. (76,78) The macular lesions heal to form a central atrophic scar. (78) Endogenous cryptococcal endophthalmitis has nonspecific ocular inflammatory signs including intraretinal hemorrhage, vascular sheathing, yellow-white chorioretinal mass or scarlike lesion. (79,80) Retinal detachment may complicate the infection. (79) The infection is usually misdiagnosed as sterile uveitis. (79) Suspicion of infection should be greater in the presence of a yellow or white chorioretinal abscess. (79,80) Coccidioidal endophthalmitis is an uncommon presentation in patients with disseminated disease. (81) Usually a severe granulomatous iridocyclitis characterized by mutton- fat keratic precipitates is present. (81) Multifocal choroiditis, typified by several, scattered, discrete yellow-white lesions measuring less than the disc diameter in size, is observed. (81) Occasionally, vascular sheathing, vitreous haze, serous retinal detachment and retinal hemorrhage may also be seen. (81) Less commonly, Histoplasma capsulatum and other dimorphic fungi have been implicated in endogenous endophthalmitis. (57) Endogenous histoplasmic endophthalmitis has been reported in several patients with disseminated systemic histoplasmosis. (82) The ocular infection may result in a granulomatous anterior uveitis. (82) Vitritis may be mild to severe. (82) The classic fundus lesion is a cream-colored or gray-white chorioretinal infiltrate, often surrounded by hemorrhage. (82) There may be associated retinal pigment epithelial alteration, indicating partial spontaneous healing. (82) The lesions may be solitary or multiple can range from less than a disc diameter to several disc diameters. (83) Histoplasmic optic neuritis has also been reported in association with the chorioretinitis. (83) The ocular findings are not specific for histoplasmic endophthalmitis, and the diagnosis should be suspected in any immunosuppressed patient living in an area endemic for histoplasmosis. (83) Rare causes of endogenous fungal endophthalmitis include Fusarium species, Mucormycosis, Paecilomyces species, Pencillium species, Bipolaris hawaiiensis, and Trichosporon beigelii. (84,85) Endophthalmitis due to systemic fungaemia is less commonly reported in East Asian countries. (57)

8. Diagnosis

The high incidence of misdiagnosis of endogenous endophthalmitis ranging from conjunctivitis, acute glaucoma or other ocular conditions should alert the ophthalmologist to make a correct diagnosis of this insidious entity. The possibility of endogenous endophthalmitis should be considered in any patient who manifests a pronounced anterior reaction that is refractory to steroid treatment. The appropriate diagnosis is necessary to start the appropriate treatment and influence dramatically the visual outcome as well as reduce the incidence of systemic complications, sometime fatal. Therefore the crucial point is diagnostic suspicion. The diagnostic algorithm should include accurate ocular and systemic history, investigation of risk factors, search source of infection, fluorescein angiography, (Fig. 12) B/A scan ocular ultrasonography, (Fig. 13) and computerized tomography of the orbit (Fig. 14) to exclude posterior involvement, and during the follow-up to monitor the adequacy of treatment, anterior aqueous tap, vitreous tap or vitrectomy, gram stain and culture of ocular and non-ocular fluids including blood, urine, cerebrospinal fluid. Organisms are cultured from ocular fluid in 36-73% of cases. (50) In many cases, prior treatment for systemic infection with intravenous antibiotics had already been instituted and this would reduce the culture positive rate from ocular fluids. A second factor resulting

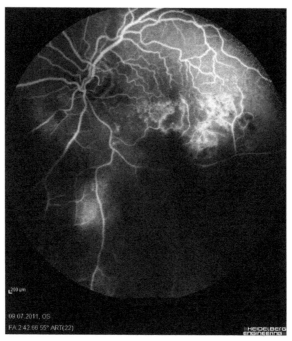

Fig. 12. Fluorescein angiography showing the areas of vascular leakage (hyperfluorescent) and the areas of retinal hemorrhage (hypofluorescent)

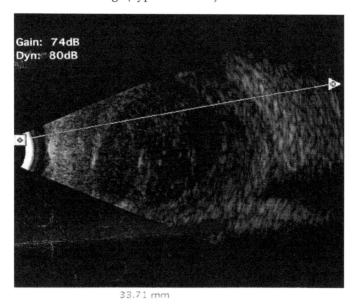

Fig. 13. B-Scan ultrasonography of the eye showing scleral thickening and dense vitreous inflammatory opacifications

in a negative culture is sampling from an inappropriate compartment within the eye. Both aqueous and vitreous cultures should be obtained unless the organism has been identified from a non-ocular source. Beyond an initial diagnostic aqueous and vitreous tap, a pars plana vitrectomy can provide additional material for culture. It should be inoculated in blood agar, chocolate agar, brain-heart infusion broth/agar, thioglycollate broth and Sabouraud agar. (50) A specimen sent for Gram stain may allow provisional categorization of the organism. Polymerase chain reaction (PCR) may allow rapid identification of organism with high sensitivity, but specificity may be a problem and facilitates for this test are not widely available. (50) In comparison with bacterial endogenous endophthalmitis, those case caused by fungi rarely have a positive blood culture. (86) Systemic fungaemia is either transient or not recognized prior to eye infection. (47) On the other hand, screening of several series of patients with candidaemia has not revealed any cases of endophthalmitis. (47) The benefit of screening lucid, asymptomatic patients thus remains doubtful at this point of time. (47,50) However, vitreous cultures will often reveal the offending organisms in these cases. (86) Vitrectomy samples are more sensitive for fungal cultures than vitreous needle biopsies. (86) The cultures must be kept at the laboratory for at least 4-6 weeks to ensure that slow-growing or fastidious fungal organisms are not missed. (86) PCR is also used as a diagnostic tool for fungal endophthalmitis. (87,88) The main advantage of PCR over conventional fungal cultures are the higher sensitivity and the rapid results. (87,88) Although PCR does not replace conventional mycologic methods, it helps to make an early differentiation between bacterial endophthalmitis and fungal endophthalmitis. (88) Candida species grow well on Sabouraud media without cycloheximide. (89) The colonies are white and pasty. (89) Aspergilli species are observed best with Grocott Methenamine Silver (GMS) or Periodic acid-Schiff (PAS) stains. (90) Aspergilli cultures are initially flat, white and filamentous. (90) Within 48 hours, conidia are produced with a concomitant change in

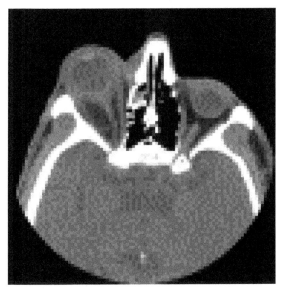

Fig. 14. Orbital tomography showing proptosis, extraocular muscle enlargement, soft tissue swelling and retrobulbar fat stranding of the left eye

pigmentation. (90) Cryptococci also grow well in Sabouraud agar. (91) It may be identified by India ink. (91) Coccidioidomycosis can be diagnosed using a 10% KOH mount and identifying endospores that contain spherules. (92)

Apart from microbiological investigation, other tests may be required according to the clinical picture. These would include complete blood cell count with differential, erythrocyte sedimentation rate, blood urea nitrogen and creatinine.

8.1 Differential diagnosis

Endogenous endophthalmitis should always be considered early in the differential diagnosis of anterior uveitis. (87) The common causes of anterior uveitis must be excluded by the usual serological tests. (87) Glaucoma, CMV retinitis, toxoplasma chorioretinitis, primary intraocular lymphoma, syphilitic chorioretinitis, autoimmune causes, malignancies, masquerade, metastatic tumors, and other infectious diseases should also be ruled out. (93) Rarely, cavernous sinus thrombosis, corneal abrasion, corneal laceration, corneal ulceration and ulcerative keratitis, globe rupture, herpes zoster ophthalmicus and vitreous hemorrhage are included in the differential diagnosis. (78,94)

9. Medical treatment

9.1 Systemic therapy

Prompt administration of antibiotic therapy is the key in the acute management of endogenous endophthalmitis. Systemic antibiotics also treat distant foci of infection and prevent continued bacteremia, thereby reducing the chances of invasion of the unaffected eye. Prolonged intravenous therapy is usually required for 2-4 weeks, until it is certain that the systemic infection is eradicated. (33) Empiric broad-spectrum antibiotic therapy with vancomycin and aminoglycoside or a third-generation cephalosporin is recommended at the highest theurapeutic doses. (33,52) Gentamycine has the coverage of gram-negative organisms including Pseudomonas aeruginosa. (25,44) It is the first choice aminoglycoside for systemic gram-negative coverage. (25,44) It has bacteriocidal activity by binding to 30S ribosomal subunit and inhibiting protein synthesis. (44) Ceftazidime is the third-generation cephalosporin with broad gram-negative coverage but decreased efficacy to gram-positive organisms. (95,96) It binds to one or more of the penicillin-binding proteins and prevent cell wall synthesis inhibiting bacterial growth. (95) Ceftriaxone is another third-generation cephalosporin is active against the resistant gram-negative organisms. (12) For Gram-positive cover, intravenous vancomycin is warranted in the view of the potential severity of the disease and consequences. (95,96) Good Gram-negative coverage is provided by third-generation cephalosporins, ciprofloxacin and aminoglycosides. (25,44) Although intravenous antibiotics can reach therapeutic concentrations in affected eyes, the use of systemic antibiotics that have good intraocular penetration and bioavailability is preferred. (97,98) In particular, aminoglycosides do not have good intraocular bioavailability when given intravenously. (44) In specific situations, certain antibiotics should be preferred. For example, bacillus infections mandate the initial use of either vancomycin or clindamycin. (41) In cases of fungal sepsis and endophthalmitis amphotericin B provides good efficacy and broad coverage. (99,100) It is fungostatic or fungocidal depending on concentration attained in body fluids. (101) It is an polyene antibiotic and it changes permeability of fungal cell membrane by binding to sterols, which causes fungal cell death as intracellular components leak out. (101) Treatment duration and total dose of intravenous drug are determined by the clinical response and the degree of systemic or non-ocular involvement. (102) Toxic side effects including renal and hepatic toxicity must be carefully monitored. (102) The penetration of amphotericin B into vitreous cavity is poor. (103) Doses of 5-10 microgram of intravitreal amphotericin is used for treatment. (103) However, retinal toxicities have also been reported in animal models at these doses. (103) The azole antibiotics are less toxic and have better ocular penetration. (104) Fluconazole and flucytosine have good intraocular penetration, but Candida species show high resitance to flucytosine. (104) Flucytosine can be used in combination with amphotericin B in cases of macular involvement and extensive inflammatory response. (100,104) Itraconazole is useful in Aspergillus and Fusarium infections. (99) A new systemic voriconazole, when administered orally or intravenously, it has good intravitreal concentrations. (100) Intravitreal administration of voriconazole is also safe without evidence of retinal toxicity with concentrations up to 25 microgram/ml. (105) The echinocandins (caspofungin, micafungin, and anidulafungin) are newer agents that exert their antifungal activity by binding D-glucan synthase, an enzyme involved in fungal cell wall synthesis. (106,107) Because mammalian cells lack a cell wall, it also represents an ideal and specific target for antifungal therapy. (106) Echinocandins exert antifungal activity against Candida and Aspergillus species. (106,107) However, they have limited penetration into the vitreous cavity so their role in the treatment of fungal endophthalmitis needs to be determined. (107)

9.2 Intravitreal therapy

Although the value of intravitreal antibiotics over and above the use of intravenous antibiotics has not been definitively established, most cases in our experience are of posterior diffuse disease and panophthalmitis which denote severe infection with extension of organisms into the vitreous. These cases should be treated aggressively as possible with both systemic and intravitreal antibiotics. In cases caused by bacteria, intravitreal injection of vancomycin 1mg/0.1ml and ceftazidime 2mg/0.1 ml provides good coverage and avoids the toxicity associated with aminoglycosides. (41,108) Repeated injections may be required since the half-life of these drugs in the vitreous cavity is short. (108) In most cases of fungal endophthalmitis, an intravitreal injection of 5-10 microgram amphotericin B is recommended. (103) Using amphotericin B in this manner avoids its numerous systemic side effects, but its potential for retinal toxicity should be noted. (103) The use of intravitreal, topical and subtenon steroids should be avoided in fungal endophthalmitis. (99) However, the use of intravitreal steroid, dexamethasone in addition to intravitreal antibiotics is recommended for suppression of inflammatory mediators released in the vitreous in bacterial endophthalmitis. (108-111) The histopathological changes of the eyes treated with intravitreal vancomycin with dexamethasone (0.4 mg/ml) had less conjunctival inflammation, mild iridocyclitis, less vitreous cells, less choroidal vasculitis and retinitis compared to antibiotic treatment alone. (109,110)

Topical steroids are also used in patients with anterior focal or diffuse endophthalmitis to reduce the number of inflammatory cells in the anterior chamber, thereby preventing the complications such as formation of synechiae and secondary glaucoma. (112-114)

Topical antibiotics are definitively indicated if keratitis develops and adjunctive therapy includes the use of cycloplegics, ocular hypotensives and topical steroids. (113,114)

9.3 Surgical treatment

The timing of and necessity for vitrectomy remains unclear in endogenous endophthalmitis. (115,116) The benefits of vitreous tap outweigh the benefits of vitrectomy for anterior focal or diffuse and posterior focal cases with endogenous endophthalmitis. (38) In general vitrectomy is indicated in cases of posterior diffuse cases with prominent vitreous involvement, and also for cases showing progressive disease despite intensive medical therapy. (116) In these cases small gauge vitrectomy is effective in clearing the vitreous from the inflammatory debris, cells and mediators. (117) Other advantage includes the possibility to have larger sample to make the diagnosis and also to deliver a therapeutic level of drug in the vitreous. (118,119) In these cases vitrectomy and intravitreal antibiotics may, however, prevent ocular atrophy or the necessity for enucleation. (119)

10. Prognosis

The visual outcome is usually good in the anterior form of endophthalmitis, differently from posterior diffuse and panophthalmitis forms. (19) The outcome of posterior diffuse endophthalmitis or panophthalmitis is frequently blindness, regardless of the treatment measures. (19) In a recent study surveying cases in Singapore over a 4-year period, 17 of 32 affected eyes ended up with no light perception. (4) In only 40% of patients with endogenous endophthalmitis vision is preserved with ability to count fingers or better. (4)

The virulence factor of the organism and age of the patient are important factors predicting outcome. (4,5) Other variables resulting in poorer outcome include severity of underlying systemic illness, misdiagnosis or delay in diagnosis, and inappropriate, inadequate or delayed treatment, low intraocular pressure, initial visual acuity of light perception, severe hypopyon and absent red reflex. (5,6) Ultrasonography negative prognostic factors are vitreous and subhyaloid opacities, choroidal and retinal detachments. (35) In general Gram-positive infections involving microbes such as Staphylococcus and Streptococcus species result in a better outcome. (112,120) However, Bacillus infections are typically rapidly progressive with a poorer prognosis. (120) Gram-negative organisms, including Klebsiella pneumonia, E. coli, P aeruginosa, often result in severe infection and a very poor prognosis. (6,12) Exceptions include Haemophilus and Neisseria, but these are uncommon causes of endogenous endophthalmitis. (121,122) Fungal endogenous endophthalmitis usually result in very poor outcomes, but those caused by Candida species can often be treated effectively if early and appropriate antifungals are used. (98,99)

11. Conclusion

Endogenous endophthalmitis continues to occur among the patients with infective endocarditis despite the continuing development of effective antibiotics. Although it is devastating, vision can sometimes be salvaged, especially if diagnosis is made early and prompt systemic therapy instituted. The role of intravitreal antibiotics and vitrectomy is not well defined but they have a definite role in cases which progress despite medical therapy and also where fungi are implicated. Future challenge ahead include the aging population and the development of new microbial antibiotic resistance. A coordinated multidisciplinary effort will be required to keep abreast of this difficult condition.

12. References

[1] Lopez J, Revilla A, Vilacosta I, et al. Multiple-valve infective endocarditis: Clinical, microbiologic, echocardiographic and prognostic profile. Medicine (Baltimore) 2011 Jun 18 (Epub ahead of print)

[2] Silverman ME, Upshaw CB Jr. Extra-cardiac manifestations of infective endocarditis and their historical descriptions. Am J Cardiol 2007;100:1802-7.

[3] Walpot J, Klazen C, blok W, et al. Embolic events in infective endocarditis: a review and report of 4 cases. Acta Clin Belg 2005;60:139-45.

[4] Ming PY, Phaik CS. Endogenous endophthalmitis SGH Proceedings 2004;13:113-20.

[5] Okada AA, Johnson RP, Liles WC, et al. Endogenous bacterial endophthalmitis: report of a ten-year prospective study. Ophthalmology 1994;101:832-8.

[6] Wong JS, Chan TK, Lee HM, et al. Endogenous bacterial endophthalmitis: an East Asian experience and a reappraisal of a severe ocular affliction. Ophthalmology 2000;107:1483-91.

[7] Lee SY, Chee SP. Group B Streptococcus endogenous endophthalmitis. Case reports and review of the literature. Ophthalmology 2002;109:1879-86.

[8] Chee SP, Ang CL. Endogenous Klebsiella endophthalmitis- a case series. Ann Acad Med Singapore 1995;24:473-8.

[9] Jain ML, Garg AK. Metastatic endophthalmitis in a patient with major burns: a rare complication. Burns 1995;21:72-3.

[10] Banerjee SN, Emori TG, Culver DH, et al. Secular trends in nosocomial primary bloodstream infections in the United States, 1980-1989. National Nosocomial Infections Surveillance System. Am J Med 1991;91:86S-89S.

[11] Chee SP, Jap A. Endogenous endophthalmitis. Current Opinion in Ophthalmology 2001;12:464-70.

[12] Yang CS, Tsai HY, Sung CS, et al. Endogenous Klebsielle endophthalmitis associated with pyogenic liver abscess. Ophthalmology 2007;114:876-80.

[13] Kiwan YA, Hayat N, Vijayaraghavan DG, et al. Infective endocarditis: A prospective study of 60 consecutive cases. Mater Med Pol 1990;22:173-5.

[14] Al-Tawfiq JA, Sufi I. Infective endocarditis at a hospital in Saudi Arabia: epidemiology, bacterial pathogens and outcome. Ann Saudi Med 2009; 29:433-6.

[15] Binder MI, Chua J, Kaiser PK, et al. Endogenous endophthalmitis. An 18-year review of culture-positive cases at a tertiary care center. Medicine (Baltimore) 2003;82:97-105.

[16] Durand ML. Bacterial endophthalmitis. Curr Infect Dis Rep 2009;11:283-8.

[17] Schiedler V, Scott IU, Flynn HW Jr, et al. Culture-proven endogenous endophthalmitis: clinical features and visual acuity outcomes. Am J Ophthalmol 2004;137:725-31.

[18] Ness T, Serr A. Diagnostics for endophthalmitis. Klin Monbl Augenheilkd 2008;225:44-9.

[19] Liang L, Lin X, Yu A, et al. The clinical analysis of endogenous endophtahlmitis. Yan Ke Xue Bao 2004,20:144-8.

[20] Greenwald MJ, Wohl LG, Sell H. Metastatic bacterial endophthalmitis: a contemporary reappraisal. Surv Ophthalmol 1986;31:81-101.

[21] Puliafito CA, Baker AS, Foster CS. Infectious endophthalmitis. Ophthalmology 1982;89:921-9.

[22] Pflugfelder CS, Flynn HW Jr. Infectious endophthalmitis. Infect Dis Clin North Am 1992;6:859-73.

[23] Davis JL, Nussenblat RB, Bachman DM, et al. Endogenous bacterial retinitis in AIDS. Am J Ophthalmol 1989;107:613-23.

[24] Margo CE, Mames RN, Guy JR. Endogenous Klebsiella endophthalmitis. Report of two cases and review of the literature. Ophthalmology 1994;101:1298-301.

[25] Tseng CY, Liu PY, Shi ZY, et al. Endogenous endophthalmitis due to Escherichia coli:case report and review. Clin Infect Dis 1996;22:1107-8.

[26] Jeng BH, Kaiser BK, Lowder CY. Retinal vasculitis and posterior pole "hypopyons" as early signs of acute bacterial endophthalmitis. Am J Ophthalmol 2001;131:800-2.

[27] Magadur-Joly G, Raffi F, Bouchut P, et al. Hematogenic bacterial endophthalmitis. A rare infection with very poor functional prognosis. Ann Med Interne (Paris) 1996;147:212-7.

[28] Molina DN, Colon M, Bermudez RH, et al. Unusual presentation of Pseudomonas aeruginosa infections: a review. Bol Asoc Med P R 1991;83:160-3.

[29] Treister G, Rothoff L, Yalon M, et al. Bilateral blindeness fron panophthalmitis in a case of bacterial endocarditis. Ann Ophthalmol 1982;14:663-4.

[30] Khan A, Okhravi N, Lightman S. The eye in systemic sepsis. Clin Med 2002;2.444-8.

[31] Ness T, Pelz K, Hansen LL. Endogenous endophtahlmitis: microorganisms, disposition and prognosis. Acta Ophthalmol Scand 2007;85:852-6.

[32] Hori J, Vega JL, Masli S. Review of ocular immune privilege in the year 2010: modifying the immune privilege of the eye. Ocul Immunol Inflamm 2010;18:325-33.

[33] Novosad BD, Callegan MC. Severe bacterial endophthalmitis: towards improving clinical outcomes. Expert Rev Ophthalmol 2010;5:689-98.

[34] Bartz-Schmidt KU, Bermig J, Kirchoff B, et al. Prognostic factors associated with the visual outcome after vitrectomy for endophthalmitis. Graefes Arch Clin Exp Ophthalmol 1996;234:S51-8.

[35] Uchio E, Ohno S. Ocular manifestations of systemic infections. Curr Opin Ophtahlmol 1999;10:452-7.

[36] Riss JM, Righini-Chossegros M, Paulo F, et al. Endogenous bacterial endophthalmitis. Report of three cases. J Fr Ophthalmol 1990;13:327-31.

[37] Hutnik CM, Nicolle DA, Munoz DG. Orbital aspergillosis. A fatal masquerader. J Neuroophthalmol 1997;17:257-61.

[38] Ho V, Ho LY, Ranchod TM, et al. Endogenous methicillin-resistant Staphylococcus aureus endophthalmitis. Retina 2011;31:596-601.

[39] Saffra NA, Desai RU, Seidmann CJ, et al. Endogenous fungal endophthalmitis after cardiac surgery. Ophthalmic Surg Lasers Imaging 2010;28:e1-3.

[40] Willermain F, Bradstreet C, Kampauridis S, et al. different presentations of ophthalmic aspergillosis. Eur J Ophthalmol 2008;18:827-30.

[41] Miller JJ, Scott IU, Flynn HW Jr, et al. Endophthalmitis caused by Bacillus species. Am J Ophthalmol 2008;145:883-8.

[42] al Hazzaa SA, Tabbara KF, Gammon JA. Pink hypopyon: a sign of Serratia marcescens endophthalmitis. Br J Ophthalmol 1992;76:764-5.

[43] Equi RA, Green WR. Endogenous Serratia marcescens endophthalmitis with dark hypopyon: case report and review. Surv Ophthalmol 2001;46:259-68.

[44] Ang LP, Lee HM, Au Eong KG, et al. Endogenous Klebsiella Endophthalmitis. Eye (Lond) 2000;14:855-60.

[45] Hauch A, Elliott D, Rao NA, et al. Dark hypopyon in Streptococcus bovis endogenous endophthalmitis: clinicopathological correlations. J Ophthalmic Inflamm Infect 2010;30:39-41.

[46] Hawkins AS, Deutsch TA. Infectious endophthalmitis. Curr Infect Dis Rep 1999;1:172-77.

[47] Bogadhi B. Fungal endogenous endophthalmitis. J Fr Ophthalmol 2011;34:40-45

[48] Kaburaki T, Takamoto M, Araki F, et al. Endogenous Candida albicans infection causing subretinal abscess. Int Ophthalmol 2010;30:203-6.

[49] Rana M, Fahad B, Abid Q. Embolic aspergillus endophthalmitis in an immunocompetent patient from aortic root aspergillus endocarditis. Mycoses 2008;51:352-3.

[50] Chung KS, Kim YK, Song YG, et al. Clinical review of endogenous endophthalmitis in Korea: a 14-year review of culture positive cases of two large hospitals. Yonsei Med J 2011,1:630-4.

[51] Hueber A, Welsandt G, Grajewski RS, et al. Fulminant endogenous anterior uveitis due to Listeria monocytogenes. Case Report Ophthalmol 2010;27:63-5.

[52] Cornut PL, Chiquet C. Endogenous bacterial endophthalmitis. J Fr Ophthlmol 2011;34:51-7.

[53] Arcieri ES, Jorge EF, de Abrea Ferreira L, et al. Bilateral endogenous endophthalmitis associated with infective endocarditis: case report. Braz J Infect Dis 2001;5:356-9.

[54] Nagelberg HP, Petashnick DE, To KW, et al. Group B streptococcal metastatic endophthalmitis. Am J Ophthalmol 1994;117:498-500.

[55] Wann SR, Liu YC, Yen MY, et al. Endogenous Escherichia coli endophthalmitis. J Formos Med Assoc 1996;95:56-60.

[56] Park SB, Searl SS, Aquavella JV, et al. Endogenous endophthalmitis caused by Escherichia coli. Ann Ophthalmol 1993;25:95-9.

[57] Durante-Mangoni E, Tripodi MF, Albisinni R, et al. Management of Gram-negative and fungal endocarditis. International Journal of Antimicrobial Agents 2010;36:S40-S45.

[58] Faraawi R, Fong IW. Escherichia coli emphysematous endophthalmitis and pyelonephritis. Case report and review of the literature. Am J Med 1988;84:636-9.

[59] Tseng CY, Yuk-Fong Liu P, Shi ZY, et al. Endogenous endophthalmitis due to Escherichia coli: Case report and Review. Clinical infectious Diseases 1996;22:1107-8.

[60] Lauridsen TK, Arpi M, Fritz-Hansen T, et al. Infectious endocarditis caused by Escherichia coli. Scand J Infect Dis 2011;43:545-6.

[61] Chen YJ, Kuo HK, Wu PC, et al. A 10-year comparison of endogenous endophthalmitis outcomes: an east Asian experience with Klebsiella pneumniae infection. Retina 2004;24:383-90.

[62] Kashani AH, Eliott D. Bilateral Klebsieela pneumoniae (k1 serotype) endogenous endophthalmitis as the presenting sign of disseminated infection. Ophthalmic Surg Lasers Imaging 2011;10:e12-4.

[63] Ramonas KM, Freilich BD. Iris abscess as an unusual presentation of endogenous endophthalmitis in a patient with bacterial endocarditis. Am J Ophthalmol 2003;135:228-9.

[64] Seles S, Lang GE. Ocular manifestations of an infectious endocarditis. Klin Monbl Augenheilkd 2007;224:606-8.

[65] McCue JD, Dreher RJ. Bilateral endophthalmitis with Streptococcus viridans endocarditis. J Maine med Assoc. 1979;70:463-5.

[66] Kobayashi K, Fujiseki Y, Takahashi K, et al. Bacterial endophthalmitis caused by B streptococcus endocarditis. Nippon Ganka Gakkai Zasshi 2006;110:199-204.

[67] Chihara S, Siccion E. Group B streptococcus endophthalmitis with endocarditis. Mayo Clin Proc 2005;80:74.

[68] Pokharel D, Doan AP, Lee AG. Group B streptococcus endogenous endophthalmitis presenting as septic arthritis and a homonymous hemianopsia due to embolic stroke. Am J Ophthalmol 2004;138:300-2.

[69] Hui M. Streptococcusanginosus bacteremia: Sutton's law. J Clin Microbiol 2005;43:6217.

[70] Hadid OH, Shah SP, Sherafat H, et al. Streptococcus anginosus-associated endogenous endophthalmitis mimicking fungal endophthalmitis. J Clin Microbiol 2005;43:4275-6.

[71] Dreier J, Vollmer T, Freytag CC, et al. Culture-negative infectious endocarditis caused by Bartonella spp.: 2 case reports and a review of the literature. Diagn Microbiol Infect Dis 2008;61:476-83.

[72] Puechal X. Whipple's disease. Rev Med Interne 2009;30:233-41.

[73] Edouard S, Raoult D. Bartonella henselae, an ubiquitous agent of proteiform zoonotic disease. Med Mal Infect 2010;40:319-30.

[74] Escher R, Roth S, Droz S, et al. Endocarditis due to Tropheryma whipplei: rapid detection, limited genetic diversity, and long-term clinical outcome in a local experience. Clin Microbiol Infect 2010;16:1213-22.

[75] Falcone M, Barzaghi N, Carosi G, et al. Candida infective endocarditis: report of 15 cases from a prospective multicenter study. Medicine (Baltimore) 200988:160-8.

[76] Rao NA, Hidayat A. a comparative clinicopathologic study of endogenous mycotic endophthalmitis: variations in clinical and histological changes in candidiasis compared to aspergillosis. Trans Am Ophthalmol Soc 2000;98:183-93.

[77] Brooks RG. Prospective study of Candida endophthalmitis in hospitalized patients with candidemia. Arch Inter Med 1989;149:226-8.

[78] Weishaar PD, Flynn HW Jr, Murray TG, et al. Endogenous aspergillus endophthalmitis: Clinical features and treatment outcomes. Ophthalmology 1998;105:57-65.

[79] Sheu SJ, Chen YC, Kuo NW, et al. Endogenous cryptococcal endophthalmitis. Ophthalmology 1998;105:377-81.

[80] Crump JR, Elner SG, Elner VM, et al. Cryptococcal endophthalmitis: case report and review. Clin Infect Dis 1992;14:1069-73.

[81] Blumenkranz MS, Stevens DA. Endogenous coccidioidal endophthalmitis. Ophthalmology 1980;87;974-84.

[82] Weingeist TA, Watzke RC. Ocular involvement by histoplasma capsulatum. Int Ophthalmol Clin 1983;23:33-47.

[83] Leung C, Farmer JP, Zoutman DE, et al. Histoplasma capsulatum endophthalmitis in southeastern Ontario. Can J Ophthalmol 2010;45:90-1.

[84] Louie T, el Baba F, Shulman M, et al. Endogenous endophthalmitis due to Fusarium: case report and review. Clin Infect Dis 1994;18:585-8.

[85] McGuire TW, Bullock JD, Bullock JD Jr, et al. Fungal endophthalmitis. An experimental study with a review of 17 human ocular cases. Arch Ophthalmol 1991;109:1289-96.

[86] Kalkancı A, Ozdek S. Ocular fungal Infections. Curr Eye Res 2011;36:179-89.

[87] Vasseneix C, Bodaghi B, Muraine M, et al. Intraocular fluids analysis for etiologic diagnosis of presumed infectious uveitis. J Fr Ophthalmol 2006;29:398-403.

[88] Harper TW, Miller D, Schiffman JC, et al. Polymerase chain reaction analysis of aqueous and vitreous specimens in the diagnosis of posterior segment infectious uveitis. Am J Ophthalmol 2009;147:140-7.

[89] Odds FC, Bernaerts R. Chromagar candida, a new differential isolation medium for presumptive isolation of clinically important candida species. Journal of Clinical Microbiology 1994;32:1923-9.

[90] Piao YS, Liu HG, Liu XJ. Significance of MUC5B antibody in differential diagnosis between Aspergillus species and Mucorales of fungal sinusitis. Zhonghua Bing Li Xue Za Zhi 2008;37:255-8.

[91] Shashikala, Kanungo R, Srinivasan S, et al. Unusual morphological forms of Cryptococcus neoformans in cerebrospinal fluid. Indian J Med Microbiol 2004;22:188-90.

[92] Sarosi GA, Lawrence JP, Smith DK, et al. Rapid diagnostic evaluation of bronchial washings in patients with suspected coccidioidomycosis. Semin Respir Infect 2001;16:238-41.

[93] Turno-Krecicka A, Misiuk-Hojlo M, Grzybowski A, et al. Early vitrectomy and diagnostic testing in severe infectious posterior uveitis and endophthalmitis. Med Sci Monit 2010;16:296-300.

[94] Heidemann DG, Trese M, Murphy SF, et al. Endogenous Listeria monocytogenes endophthalmitis presenting as keratouveitis. Cornea 1990;9:179-80.

[95] Connell PP, O'Neill EC, Fabiyni D, et al. Endogenous endophthalmitis: 10-year experience at a tertiary referral center. Eye (Lond) 2011;25:66-72.

[96] Torii H, Miyata H, Sugisaka E, et al. Bilateral endophthalmitis in a patient with bacterial meningitis caused by Streptococcus pneumonia. Ophthalmologica 2008;222:357-9.

[97] Ang M, Jap A, Chee SP. Prognostic factors and outcomes in endogenous Klebsiella pneumonia endophthalmitis. Am J Ophthalmol 2011;151:338-44.

[98] Connell PP, O'Neill EC, Amirul Islam FM, et al. Endogenous endophthalmitis associated with intravenous drug abuse: seven-year experience at a tertiary referral center. Retina 2010;30:1721-5.

[99] Chakrabarti A, Shivaprakash MR, Singh R, et al. Fungal endophthalmitis: Fourteen years' experience from a center in India. Retina 2008;28:1400-7.

[100] Riddell J 4th, Corner GM, Kaufmann CA. Treatment of endogenous fungal endophthalmitis: focus on new antifungal agents. Clin Infect Dis 2011;52:648-53.

[101] Goldblum D, Rohrer K, Frueh BE, et al. Ocular distribution of intravenously administered lipid formulations of amphotericin B in a rabbit model. Antimic Agents Chemother 2002;46:3719-23.

[102] Narendran N, Balasubramaniam B, Johnson E, et al. Five-year retrospective review of guideline-based management of fungal endophthalmitis. Acta Ophthalmol 2008;86:525-32.

[103] Payne JF, Keenum DG, Sternberg P Jr, et al. Concentrated intravitreal amphotericin B in fungal endophthalmitis. Arch Ophthalmol 2010;128;1546-50.

[104] Annamalai T, Fong KC, Choo MM. Intravenous fluconazole for bilateral endogenous Candida endophthalmitis. J Ocul Phramacol Ther 2011;27:105-7.

[105] Funakoshi Y, Yakushijin K, Matsuoka H, et al. Fungal endophthalmitis successfully treated with intravitreal voriconazole injection. Intern Med 2011;50:941.

[106] Mora-Duarte J, Betts R, Rotstein C, et al. Comparision of capsofungin and amphotericin B for invasive candidiasis. N Eng J Med 2002;347:2020-9.

[107] Gauthier GM, Nork TM, Prince R, et al. Subtheurapeutic ocular penetration of capsofungin and associated treatment failure in candida albicans endophthalmitis. Clin Inf Dis 2005;41:27-8.

[108] Mehta S, Armstrong BK, Kim SJ et al. Long-term potency, sterility and stability of vancomycin, ceftazidime and moxifloxacin for treatment of bacterial endophthalmitis. Retina 2011;Feb 23 (Epub ahead of print)

[109] Albrecht E, Richards JC, Polock T, et al. Adjunctive use of intravitreal dexamethasone in presumed bacterial endophthalmitis: a randomised trial. Br J Ophthalmol 2011;Feb 2 (Epub ahead of print)

[110] Liu F, Kwok AK, Cheung BM. The efficacy of intravitreal vancomycin and dexamethasone in the treatment of experimental bacillus cereus endophtahlmitis. Curr Eye Res 2008;33:761-8.

[111] Ermis SS, Cetinkaya Z, Kıyıcı H, et al. Effects of intravitreal moxifloxacin and dexamethasone in experimental Staphylococcus endophthalmitis. Curr Eye Res 2007;32:337-44.

[112] Nentwich MM, Kampik A, de Kaspar HM. Chronic endogenous endophthalmitis. Klin Monbl Augenheilkd 2008;225:929-33.

[113] Pavesio CE, Decory HH. Treatment of ocular inflammatory conditions with loteprednol etabonate. Br J Ophthalmol 2008;92:455-9.

[114] Smith A, Pennefather PM, Kaye SB, et al. Fluoroquinolones: place in ocular therapy. Drugs 2001;61:747-61.

[115] Laube T, Akgül H, Brockmann C, et al. Endogenous bacterial endophthalmitis: a retrospective study in 22 consecutive cases. Klin Monbl Augenheilkd 2004;221:101-8.

[116] Maguire JL. Postoperative endophthalmitis: optimal management and the role and timing of vitrectomy surgery. Eye (London) 2008;22:1290-300.

[117] Thompson JT. Advantages and limitations of small gauge vitrectomy. Surv Ophthalmol 2011;56:162-72.

[118] Wen X, Zhong K, Wang Z, et al. Vitrectomy combined with intravitreal injection of drugs for the management of advanced suppurative endophthalmitis. Yan Ke Xue Bao 1992;8:164-8.

[119] Yarng SS, Hsieh CC, Chen TL. Vitrectomy for endogenous Klebsiella pneumonia endophthalmitis with massive subretinal abscess. Ophthalmic Surg Lasers 1997;128:147-50.

[120] Vahey JB, Flynn HW Jr. Results in the management of Bacillus endophthalmitis. 1991;22:681-6.

[121] Sullivan P, Clark WL, Kaiser PK. Bilateral endogenous endophthalmitis caused by HACEK microorganism. Am J Ophthalmol 2002;133:144-5.

[122] Balaskas K, Potamitou D. Endogenous endophthalmitis secondary to bacterial meningitis from Neissereia meningitides: a case report and review of the literature. Cases J 2009;2:149.

Permissions

The contributors of this book come from diverse backgrounds, making this book a truly international effort. This book will bring forth new frontiers with its revolutionizing research information and detailed analysis of the nascent developments around the world.

We would like to thank Prof. Dr. Francisco Ramón Breijo-Márquez, for lending his expertise to make the book truly unique. He has played a crucial role in the development of this book. Without his invaluable contribution this book wouldn't have been possible. He has made vital efforts to compile up to date information on the varied aspects of this subject to make this book a valuable addition to the collection of many professionals and students.

This book was conceptualized with the vision of imparting up-to-date information and advanced data in this field. To ensure the same, a matchless editorial board was set up. Every individual on the board went through rigorous rounds of assessment to prove their worth. After which they invested a large part of their time researching and compiling the most relevant data for our readers. Conferences and sessions were held from time to time between the editorial board and the contributing authors to present the data in the most comprehensible form. The editorial team has worked tirelessly to provide valuable and valid information to help people across the globe.

Every chapter published in this book has been scrutinized by our experts. Their significance has been extensively debated. The topics covered herein carry significant findings which will fuel the growth of the discipline. They may even be implemented as practical applications or may be referred to as a beginning point for another development. Chapters in this book were first published by InTech; hereby published with permission under the Creative Commons Attribution License or equivalent.

The editorial board has been involved in producing this book since its inception. They have spent rigorous hours researching and exploring the diverse topics which have resulted in the successful publishing of this book. They have passed on their knowledge of decades through this book. To expedite this challenging task, the publisher supported the team at every step. A small team of assistant editors was also appointed to further simplify the editing procedure and attain best results for the readers.

Our editorial team has been hand-picked from every corner of the world. Their multi-ethnicity adds dynamic inputs to the discussions which result in innovative outcomes. These outcomes are then further discussed with the researchers and contributors who give their valuable feedback and opinion regarding the same. The feedback is then collaborated with the researches and they are edited in a comprehensive manner to aid the understanding of the subject.

Apart from the editorial board, the designing team has also invested a significant amount of their time in understanding the subject and creating the most relevant covers. They scrutinized every image to scout for the most suitable representation of the subject and create an appropriate cover for the book.

The publishing team has been involved in this book since its early stages. They were actively engaged in every process, be it collecting the data, connecting with the contributors or procuring relevant information. The team has been an ardent support to the editorial, designing and production team. Their endless efforts to recruit the best for this project, has resulted in the accomplishment of this book. They are a veteran in the field of academics and their pool of knowledge is as vast as their experience in printing. Their expertise and guidance has proved useful at every step. Their uncompromising quality standards have made this book an exceptional effort. Their encouragement from time to time has been an inspiration for everyone.

The publisher and the editorial board hope that this book will prove to be a valuable piece of knowledge for researchers, students, practitioners and scholars across the globe.

List of Contributors

Breijo-Marquez and M. Pardo Rios
Commemorative Hospital, Boston, Massachusetts, USA
Catholic University, Murcia, Spain

Inmaculada Tomás-Carmona
Santiago de Compostela University, Spain

M. Álvarez-Fernández
Xeral-Cíes Hospital (Vigo), Spain

Steven W. Kerrigan and Dermot Cox
Royal College of Surgeons in Ireland, Dublin, Ireland

Lucy Miller and Jim George
Department of Medicine for the Elderly, Cumberland Infirmary, Carlisle, U.K.

Cédric Jacqueline, Gilles Amador, Eric Batard, Virginie Le Mabecque, Gilles Potel and Jocelyne Caillon
Université de Nantes, Faculté de Médecine, UPRES EA 3826, Nantes, France

Yuko Ohara-Nemoto and Takayuki K. Nemoto
Department of Oral Molecular Biology, Course of Medical and Dental Sciences, Nagasaki University Graduate School of Biomedical Sciences, Japan

Shigenobu Kimura
Division of Molecular Microbiology, Department of Microbiology, Iwate Medical University, Japan

C. Prados, C. Carpio, A. Santiago, I. Silva and R. Álvarez-Sala
Pulmonology Service, La Paz University Hospital, Autónoma University, Madrid, Spain

Ozlem Sahin
Middle East Technical University Health Sciences Department of Ophthalmology, Ankara, Turkey